Surgical Exposures in Orthopaedics

STANLEY HOPPENFELD, M.D.

Associate Clinical Professor of Orthopaedic Surgery,
Albert Einstein College of Medicine;

Attending Physician, Hospital of the Albert Einstein College of Medicine,
Montefiore Hospital and Misericordia Hospital;

Associate Attending, Orthopaedic Institute of the Hospital for Joint Diseases
and Westchester County Medical Center

PIET deBOER, M.A., F.R.C.S.

Senior Registrar, St. Thomas Hospital, London, England

IN
COLLABORATION
WITH
RICHARD HUTTON

ILLUSTRATED
BY
HUGH A. THOMAS

Surgical Exposures in Orthopaedics

THE ANATOMIC APPROACH

J. B. LIPPINCOTT COMPANY

PHILADELPHIA

London   Mexico City

New York   St. Louis

São Paulo   Sydney

Sponsoring Editor: Richard Winters
Manuscript Editor: Leslie E. Hoeltzel
Indexer: Sandra King
Art Director: Maria S. Karkucinski
Designer: Arlene Putterman
Production Coordinator: Susan A. Caldwell
Compositor: Ruttle, Shaw & Wetherill, Inc.
Printer/Binder: Halliday Lithograph

6 5 4 3

Library of Congress Cataloging in Publication Data

Hoppenfeld, Stanley.
    Surgical exposures in orthopaedics.

    Bibliography: p.
    Includes index.
    1. Orthopedic surgery.   2. Anatomy, Surgical and
topographical.   I. deBoer, Piet.   II. Title.
RD732.H66   1984   617'.3   83-16272
ISBN 0-397-50597-3

Dedication

To my wife Norma,
my children
Jon-David, Robert, and Stephen,
and my parents Agatha and David,
all in their own special way
have made my life full
and made this book possible.

S.H.

To Jill.
P. deB.

Preface

It has often been said that successful orthopaedic procedures are based on a simple principle: "Get to bone and stay there." *Surgical Exposures in Orthopaedics: The Anatomic Approach*, the product of an anatomy course for orthopaedic surgeons that has been run at the Albert Einstein College of Medicine for the past 15 years, expands on the principle. The book explains the techniques of commonly used orthopaedic approaches and relates the regional anatomy of the area relevant to the approach.

Safety in surgery depends on knowledge of anatomy and technical skill. The two go hand in hand; one is useless without the other. Surgical skill can be learned only by practical experience under expert supervision. But the knowledge that underlies it must come from both book and dissection.

Structurally, this book is divided into 11 chapters, each dealing with a particular area of the body. The most commonly performed approaches are described; we have omitted approaches designed only for one specific procedure—they are best understood in the original papers of those who first described them. Nevertheless, the vast majority of orthopaedic procedures can be safely and successfully accomplished through the approaches we have included.

Orthopaedics is a rapidly evolving field. New procedures are appearing at a prodigious rate; some are discarded in a comparatively short time. Thus, any book that concerns itself with the specifics of operative surgery inevitably becomes dated, sometimes even before publication. To avoid this problem, we have concentrated on getting to the bone or joint concerned, and not on what to do after. When applicable, we have included references to individual surgical procedures but without incorporating their details into our textbook.

The key to *Surgical Exposures in Orthopaedics* is a consistent organization throughout (*see* Table 1). Each approach is explained; then the relevant surgical anatomy of the area is discussed. When one or more approaches share anatomy, they are grouped together, with the relevant anatomical section at the end. The idea is for the surgeon to read the approach and anatomy sections together before attempting a given procedure, because once the anatomical principles of a procedure are fully understood, the logic of an approach becomes clear.

SURGICAL APPROACHES

The crucial element in successful surgical approaches is exploiting *internervous planes.* These planes lie between muscles—muscles supplied by different nerves. Internervous planes are helpful mainly because they can be used along their entire length without either of the muscles involved being denervated. These approaches can generally be extended to expose adjacent structures. Virtually all the classic *extensile* approaches to bone use internervous planes—a concept first described by A. K. Henry, who believed that if the key to operative surgery is surgical anatomy, then the key to surgical anatomy is the internervous plane.

The approach sections are structured as follows.

The introduction to each approach describes indications and points out the major advantages or disadvantages of the proposed surgery. Significant dangers are also outlined in this section.

The *position of the patient* is critical to clear, full exposures, as well as to the comfort of the operating surgeon.

Surgical *landmarks* form the basis for any incision; they are described with instructions on how to find them. The *incision* follows these key landmarks. Although the incisions described are generally straight, many

---

TABLE 1. CHAPTER OUTLINE

I. Surgical Approach
(Introduction)
Position of Patient on Operating Table
Landmarks and Incision
Internervous Plane
Superficial Surgical Dissection
Deep Surgical Dissection
Dangers
How to Enlarge the Approach
Local Measures
Extensile Measures

II. Applied Surgical Anatomy
Overview
Landmarks and Incision
Superficial Surgical Dissection and Its Dangers
Deep Surgical Dissection and Its Dangers
Special Anatomical Points

---

surgeons prefer to use curved or zigzag incisions because they heal with less tension than do equivalent straight incisions.

The approaches often allow exposure of the whole length of a bone; usually, only part of an exposure is required for any given operation.

The surgical dissection has been divided into *superficial* and *deep surgical dissections* for teaching purposes to reinforce the concept that each layer must be developed fully before the next layer is dissected. Adequate exposure depends on a systematic and deliberate technique that exploits each plane completely before deeper dissection begins.

The *dangers* of each approach are listed under four headings: nerves, vessels, muscles and tendons, and special points. The dangers are described, along with how to avoid them.

The approach section concludes with a description of *how to enlarge the approach*. All too often, the suregon discovers that the incised exposure is inadequate. There are two ways in which the exposure can be enlarged: *Local measures* include extending skin incisions, repositioning retractors, detaching muscles, or even adjusting the light source; and *extensile measures* are ways in which an approach can be extended to include adjacent bony structures. In approaches through internervous planes, extensile measures may permit the exposure of the entire length of the bone.

ANATOMICAL SECTIONS

The anatomy of each approach begins with a brief overview of the muscular anatomy, along with the arrangement of the neurovascular structures.

The anatomy of the *landmarks* relates these structures to their surroundings. The anatomy of the *skin incision* describes the angle between the incision and the natural lines of skin cleavage first described by Langer—a relationship that may influence the size and prominence of the resultant scar. Nevertheless, the site of a skin incision must be determined largely by safety and effectiveness and not by cosmetic considerations. Skin incisions generally avoid cutting major cutaneous nerves; where they might, the danger is clearly stated.

The *anatomy of the superficial and deep surgical dissection* discusses the regional anatomy encountered during the approaches—not only the anatomy of the plane to be used but also that of adjacent structures that may appear if the surgeon strays out of plane. Perhaps the greatest value of knowing topographical anatomy is in cases of trauma, where the surgeon may explore wounds with confidence, aware of the potential dangers created by any given wound. Relevant clinical information on the anatomical structures is offered, but a comprehensive clinical picture is beyond the scope of this book. The origins, insertions, actions, and nerve supplies of relevant muscles are listed in legends under the muscles' illustrations.

The anatomical and surgical illustrations are drawn from the surgeon's point of view whenever possible, with the patient on the operating table, so that the surgeon can see exactly how the approach must look when he operates.

The anatomical terms used in *Surgical Exposures in Orthopaedics* are generally those used in modern anatomical textbooks. Terms now in orthopaedic usage sometimes differ from them; when that occurs (for instance, with the flexor retinaculum/transverse carpal ligament), both terms are given. Variation also occurs in usage on either side of the Atlantic; we have used those terms on which the authors (one American and one English) have reached consensus.

It has been said that all of orthopaedic surgical approaches can be reduced to one line: "Avoid cutting round structures." This book has been written to tell you how.

Stanley Hoppenfeld, M.D.
Piet deBoer, M.A., F.R.C.S.

Acknowledgments

This book reflects the accumulated experience of many people over many decades. We should like to thank those in particular who helped us during the writing of this book.

To RICHARD HUTTON,
my long-term friend and editor, who adds organization and reality to our writings. His love of the English language is reflected in this book.

To HUGH THOMAS,
my long-term friend and medical illustrator, who added clarity to the book by his imaginative original illustrations, which reflect anatomic knowledge and clinical detail. In preparing the artwork for *Surgical Exposures in Orthopaedics: The Anatomic Approach,* he managed to draw beautifully on two continents.

To RAY COOMARASWAMY, M.D.,
for his help and guidance in writing the transabdominal and thoracotomy approaches to the spine.

To DAVID M. HIRSH, M.D.,
for his detailed, expert review of the chapter on the hip and for his guidance in its presentation and clinical details.

To BARNARD KLEIGER, M.D.,
for reviewing the chapters on the tibia and fibula and on the foot and ankle. He has been a source of inspiration to us during these years.

To ROY KULICK, M.D.,
for reviewing the chapter on the hand several times and for giving it that little extra to help its clinical tone.

To MARTIN LEVY, M.D.,
for his multiple reviews of the chapter on the knee for his valuable suggestions and clarity of thought.

To ERIC RADIN, M.D.,
for reviewing parts of our book in its early stages, encouraging us, and making valuable suggestions.

To ARTHUR SADLER, M.D.,
for his review of the chapter on the femur.

To LEONARD SEIMON, M.D.,
for reviewing the medial approach to the hip and sharing his unusual
surgical experiences with us.

To JERRY SOSLER, M.D.,
for demonstrating and reviewing the retroperitoneal approach to the spine
and his positive suggestions.

To MORTON SPINNER, M.D.,
for reviewing the chapters on the elbow and forearm, helping us with
clinical details, and for sharing a lifetime of clinical and surgical experience.

To KEITH WATSON, M.D.,
for reviewing the chapter on the shoulder.

To the BRITISH FELLOWS,
who visit the Albert Einstein College of Medicine from St. Thomas
Hospital in England each year. Each has made a major contribution to the
educational program and to our Anatomy course: *Clive Whaley, Robert
Jackson, David Gruber-Lee, David Reynolds, Roger Weeks, Fred Heatley,
Peter Johnson, Richard Foster, Kenneth Walker, Maldwyn Griffith, John
Patrick, Paul Allen, Paul Evans, Robert Johnson, Martin Knight, Rober
Simonis,* and *David Dempster.*

To the Anatomy Department of the Albert Einstein College of Medicine—
in particular

To FRANCE BAKER-COHEN,
who has worked closely with us in establishing the course each year,

and to MICHAEL D'ALESSANDRO,
who has kept the rooms and cadaver material for us.

To DR. M. BULL,
DR. E. M. CHISHOLM,
and the Examiners of the primary fellowship in London, who convinced me
that topographical anatomy was worth learning.

To RONALD FURLONG,
ERIC DENMAN,
and DAVID REYNOLDS,
for their efforts in teaching me and others operative surgery.

To the operating staff and technicians of Princess Margaret Hospital,
Swindon and St. Thomas Hospital, London—and especially

JIM LOVEGROVE,
for making surgery possible.

To ALAN APLEY,
not only for providing the model for teaching, but also for writing a book
that teaches.

To PROFESSOR KINMONTH,
FRED HEATLEY,
MALCOLM MORRISON,
and JOHN WILKINSON,
for their generous help during my own orthopaedic training.

To the fellow physicians who have participated in teaching the Anatomy course over these many years: *Uriel Adar, M.D., Russell Anderson, M.D., Mel Adler, M.D., Martin Barschi, M.D., Robert Dennis, M.D., Michael DiStefano, M.D., Henry Ergas, M.D., Aziz Eshraghi, M.D., Madgi Gabriel, M.D., Ralph Ger, M.D., Ed Habermann, M.D., Armen Haig, M.D., Steve Harwin, M.D., John Katonah, M.D., Ray Koval, M.D., Luc Lapommaray, M.D., Al Larkins, M.D., Mark Lazansky, M.D., Shelly Manspeizer, M.D., Mel Manin, M.D., David Mendes, M.D., Basil Preefer, M.D., Leela Rangaswamy, M.D., Ira Rochelle, M.D., Art Sadler, M.D., Jerry Sallis, M.D., Eli Sedlin, M.D., Lenny Seimon, M.D., Dick Selznick, M.D., Ken Seslowe, M.D., Rashmi Sheth, M.D., Bob Shultz, M.D., Richard Seigel, M.D., Norman Silver, M.D., Irvin Spira, M.D., Moe Spzorn, M.D., Richard Stern, M.D., Jacob Teladano, M.D., Alan Weisel, M.D., and Charles Weiss, M.D.*

To the residents who have participated in the Orthopaedic Anatomy course at the "Einstein," who have been a continual course of stimulation and inspiration.

To MURIEL CHALEFF,
who spent many hours helping to organize the Orthopaedic Anatomy course at the Albert Einstein College of Medicine. We owe her a great debt of gratitude for the kindness she has shown.

To LEON STRONG,
my first Professor of Anatomy in Medical School for a stimulating introduction to anatomy.

To EMANUEL KAPLAN, M.D.,
whose great fund of anatomy and comparative anatomy was passed on to many of us while we were residents.

To HERMAN ROBBINS, M.D.,
for his professional support and teaching of anatomy during the many sessions held in the library of the old Hospital for Joint Diseases.

To DR. and MRS. N. A. SHORE,
my long-term friends, who have had a positive effect on my medical writings and clinical practice.

To MR. ABRAHAM IRVINGS,
my long-term friend and accountant, who kept the financial records, helping to make this book possible.

To FRANK FERRIERI,
my long-term friend, in appreciation of his help.

To MARY KEARNEY,
my secretary, for help in communicating with the J. B. Lippincott Company and mailing and calling, and calling, and calling!

To our secretarial staff, CAMILLE MUSTO and MARY ANN BECCHETTI, who took hours out of their busy schedules to type, retype, retype, and retype the text until it was perfect.

To the professional staff at the J. B. Lippincott Company, for their help in producing this book. Special thanks to *Richard Winters,* Associate Editor, *Susan Caldwell,* Production Editor, *Deborah Althen Finch,* Director of the Production Services Group, *Tina Rebane,* Production Supervisor,

Pamela Fried, Index Editor, *Terry Norman,* Medical Copy Editor, *Leslie E. Hoeltzel,* Manuscript Editor, and *Maria Karkucinski,* Art Director, for giving form and shape to the book, and to *J. Stuart Freeman, Jr.,* Chief Medical Editor, who has befriended me over these years and has been a source of positive suggestions and inspiration.

Contents

4   The Forearm   109

5   The Wrist and Hand   141

6 The Spine   209

7 The Hip   301

8 The Femur   357

9 The Knee   389

10 The Tibia and Fibula   443

11 The Foot and Ankle   469

Index   531

Introduction: Orthopaedic Surgical Technique

Surgical technique in orthopaedics varies from surgeon to surgeon; the more experienced the surgeon, the fewer instruments he uses and the simpler his technique becomes. Certain principles, however, remain constant. They are listed below as they apply to each surgical section.

The *position of the patient* is fundamental to any approach; it is always worth taking time to ensure that the patient is in the best position and that he is secured so that he cannot move during the procedure. Operating tables are well padded, but certain bony prominences—such as the head of the fibula and greater trochanter—are not. These prominences must always be padded adequately to prevent skin breakdown and nerve entrapment during surgery. Patients who are prone must have suitable padding placed under their pelvis, chest, head, and nose to allow respiration during surgery. Many different systems ensure adequate ventilation of the patient; bolsters placed longitudinally under the side of the patient are probably the best. Ventilation of the prone patient must be adequate before surgery, since repositioning of the patient during surgery is difficult and almost inevitably contaminates the sterile field.

The surgeon should be comfortable during surgery, with the patient placed at the correct height for the surgeon's size or the table low enough to allow him to operate sitting down.

In surgery on the limbs, a tourniquet is often used to create a bloodless field, making identification of vital structures easier and expediting surgery.

To apply the tourniquet, empty the limb of blood, either by elevating it for 3 to 5 minutes or by applying a soft rubber compression bandage. The tourniquet should be padded with a soft dressing to prevent the wrinkles (and blisters) that inevitably occur when the skin is pinched. The tourniquet may be applied to the upper arm or thigh. Both of these areas are well muscled; the major nerves are protected from compression of the tourniquet. The inflated pressure of the tourniquet should be about 275 mm Hg in the upper limb and 450 mm Hg in the lower limb, depending on the circumference of the limb. Test the tourniquet by inflating it *before* applying it to the patient. In children, inflate the tourniquet to 50% above their systolic pressure. In hypertensive patients, inflate it 50% more than their systolic pressure. Finally, do not leave the tourniquet inflated for longer than 1 hour in the upper limb and 1½ hours in the lower limb to minimize risk; do not use tourniquets when the peripheral circulation of the patient is suspect or in the presence of sickle cell disease.

Partial exsanguination of the limb, which can be achieved after 2 minutes of elevation, leaves blood in the venous structures. It makes for a bloodier field during surgery but does make it easier to identify neurovascular bundles—something of immense value in, for example, lateral meniscectomy, where it is safer to identify and to coagulate the lateral inferior geniculate artery than to cut it accidentally, learning about it only after the tourniquet has been deflated. Deflate the tourniquet before closure to identify and to coagulate major bleeding points.

The *landmarks* are critical to the planning of any incision. It is often convenient to mark them on the skin with methylene blue to ensure that the skin incision lines up with them.

All skin incisions heal with the formation of scar tissue, which contracts with time. For this reason, skin incisions should not cross flexion creases at 90°; cutting perpendicular to flexion creases can cause contractures to develop over the involved joints. That is why incisions that cross major flexion creases are usually curved to traverse the crease at about 60°.

The techniques of the *superficial and deep surgical* dissections are the province of practical experience, not book knowledge. However, two techniques are frequently referred to in the book.

First, *subperiosteal dissection* protects vital structures that lie near the bone, helping to prevent their damage by instruments. The rule holds true, but vital structures often lie on the periosteum itself: The posterior interosseous nerve, for instance, lies on the periosteum neck of the radius, the radial nerve on the back of the humerus. In these cases, subperiosteal dissection *must* be strictly *subperiosteal,* something that may not be possible if the periosteum is damaged in cases of fracture. The periosteum normally detaches easily from the bone except at sites of muscle or ligament attachments, where it may adhere strongly. Blunt dissection may be difficult or impossible at sites of insertions. Note that the periosteum of children is thicker than that of adults, more easily defined, and less adherent to bone.

The second technique is that of detaching muscle from bone. Remember to strip *into* the *acute angle* that fibers make with the bone to which they attach. This is perhaps clearest in the fibula: To detach the peroneal muscles, pass an elevator from distal to proximal; to detach the interosseous membrane, where fibers run in a different direction, strip from proximal to distal.

Exposures can be improved in two ways. *Local measures* enhance the immediate exposure. *Extensile measures* allow the surgeon to expose adjacent bony structures. It is vital to appreciate that not all approaches are extensile: Specialized approaches should be used only in cases where the pathology is accurately pinpointed and where the surgeon does not have to expose any adjacent structures. Inadequate exposure is one of the most common causes of surgical failure. If the surgeon is in difficulty, one of the first things he should try is to improve the exposure either by local or by extensile means.

Surgical Exposures in Orthopaedics

1

The Shoulder

The shoulder is the most mobile joint in the body. It is surrounded by two sleeves of muscle: The outer sleeve is the deltoid muscle; the inner sleeve, the rotator cuff, is critical for the stability of the joint. The two most common pathologies that necessitate surgery are instability, such as recurrent anterior dislocation of the shoulder (see Fig. 1-26A and B), and degenerative lesions of the rotator cuff.

Three approaches are described: anterior, lateral, and posterior. Of these, the anterior approach is the "workhorse" incision of the shoulder, giving excellent exposure of both the joint and its anterior coverings. The lateral incision gives far more limited access to the upper end of the humerus, and the posterior incision, rarely used, is effective in treating recurrent posterior dislocations.

The surgical anatomy of the area is divided into three sections: anterior, lateral, and posterior. Each is found immediately after its respective operative section.

ANTERIOR APPROACH

The anterior approach offers a good wide exposure of the shoulder joint, allowing repairs of its anterior, inferior, and superior coverings to be carried out. Among its many uses, the anterior approach permits the following:

1. Reconstruction of recurrent dislocations[1-6]
2. Drainage of sepsis
3. Biopsy and excision of tumors
4. Repair of the tendon of the long head of the biceps[7]
5. Shoulder arthroplasties, which are usually inserted through modified anterior incisions[8]

The anterior approach is notorious for the amount of bleeding from skin and subcutaneous tissues that occurs during superficial dissection. The bleeding must be controlled before the deeper layers are dissected. Failure to do so may obscure important anatomical structures and endanger their integrity.

POSITION OF PATIENT

Place the patient in a supine position on the operating table. Wedge a sandbag under the spine and the medial border of the scapula to push the affected side forward while allowing the arm to fall backward, opening up the front of the joint (Fig. 1-1). Elevate the head of the table 30° to 45° to reduce venous pressure—to reduce bleeding—and to allow the blood to drain away from the operative field during surgery. If a headrest is used, make sure that it is properly padded to prevent a pressure sore on the occiput.

LANDMARKS AND INCISION

Landmarks

CORACOID PROCESS. At the deepest point in the clavicular concavity, drop your fingers distally about 1 inch from the anterior edge of the clavicle and press laterally and posteriorly in an oblique line until you feel the coracoid process. The process faces anterolaterally; because it lies deep under the cover of the pectoralis major, it can only be felt by firm palpation.

DELTOPECTORAL GROOVE. The groove is easier to see than to feel, especially in thin patients. The cephalic vein, which runs in the groove, is sometimes visible.

Incisions

The anterior aspect of the shoulder can be approached through either of two skin incisions.

ANTERIOR INCISION. Make a 10-cm to 15-cm straight incision, following the line of the delto-

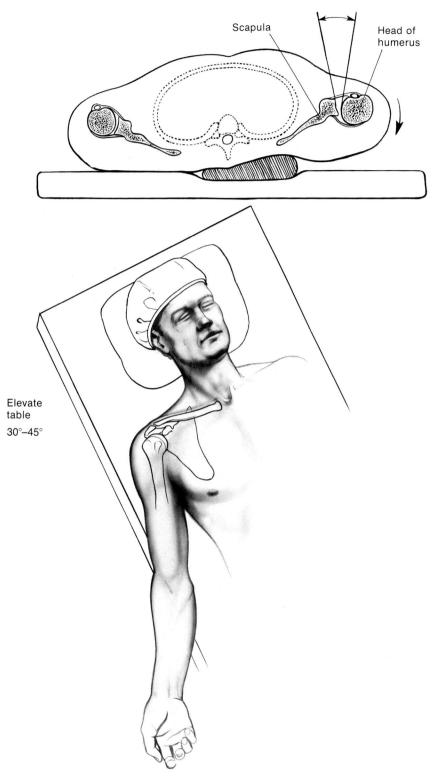

FIG. 1-1. Position of the patient for the anterior approach to the shoulder. Elevate the table to 45°. A sandbag under the spine at the medial end of the scapula will allow the shoulder to rotate externally and open the anterior part of the joint.

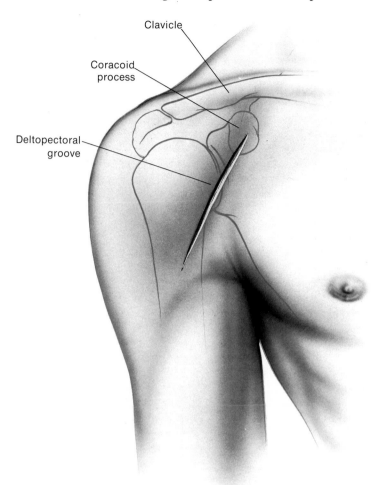

Clavicle

Coracoid process

Deltopectoral groove

FIG. 1-2. Make a straight incision in the deltopectoral groove, starting at the level of the coracoid process.

pectoral groove. The incision should begin just above the coracoid process (Fig. 1-2).

AXILLARY INCISION. With the patient supine, abduct the shoulder 90° and externally rotate it. Mark the anterior axillary skin fold with a sterile pen. Make a vertical incision 8 cm to 10 cm long, starting at the midpoint of the anterior axillary fold and extending posteriorly into the axilla.[9] Undermine the skin flaps extensively with your finger, especially superiorly in the area of the deltopectoral groove, using the cephalic vein as a guide to ensure that you are in the correct vertical plane. Retract the skin flaps upward and laterally so that the incision comes to lie over the delto-pectoral groove (Figs. 1-3 and 1-4).

The axillary incision has an extreme cosmetic advantage over the anterior incision, both because it is hidden in the axilla and because the resulting scar is covered by hair. In addition, the suture line remains free from tension while it heals; the scar thus has little opportunity to spread. (The only time that this incision may be contraindicated is when, in extremely muscular patients, the skin flaps cannot be moved enough to allow adequate exposure of the muscular structures that lie in front of the shoulder.) If you cannot get adequate exposure through the axillary incision, extend it superiorly into the deltopectoral groove.

INTERNERVOUS PLANE

The internervous plane lies between the *deltoid muscle*, supplied by the axillary nerve, and the *pectoralis major*, supplied by the medial and lateral pectoral nerves (Fig. 1-5).

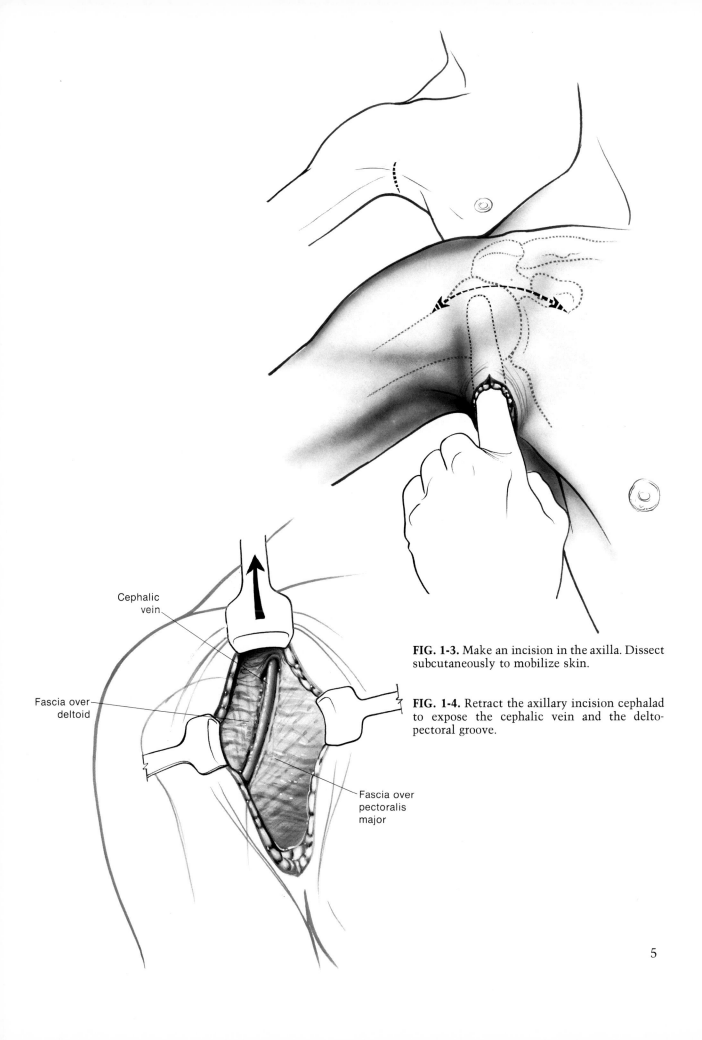

Cephalic vein

Fascia over deltoid

Fascia over pectoralis major

FIG. 1-3. Make an incision in the axilla. Dissect subcutaneously to mobilize skin.

FIG. 1-4. Retract the axillary incision cephalad to expose the cephalic vein and the delto-pectoral groove.

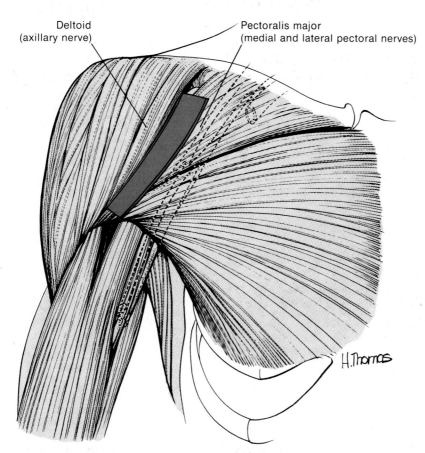

Deltoid
(axillary nerve)

Pectoralis major
(medial and lateral pectoral nerves)

FIG. 1-5. The internervous plane lies between the deltoid muscle (axillary nerve) and the pectoralis major muscle (medial and lateral pectoral nerves).

SUPERFICIAL SURGICAL DISSECTION

Find the deltopectoral groove, with its cephalic vein (Fig. 1-6). Retract the pectoralis major medially and the deltoid laterally, splitting the two muscles apart. The vein may be retracted either medially or laterally. Taking a small cuff of deltoid with the vein may reduce the number of bleeding tributaries that require ligation but leaves a small amount of denervated muscle. For that reason, it is not recommended for routine use.

DEEP SURGICAL DISSECTION

The short head of the biceps (musculocutaneous nerve) and the coracobrachialis (musculocutaneous nerve) must be displaced medially before you gain access to the anterior aspect of the shoulder joint. Simple medial retraction after division of the overlying fascia may be enough for procedures like the Magnuson-Stack subscapularis tendon advancement,[3] or the Putti-Platt subscapularis[2] and capsule imbrication, but if more exposure is necessary, the two muscles can be detached from

the coracoid process. To release them, detach the tip of the coracoid process with an osteotome. You can replace the bone later either with a screw or with sutures. If you use a screw, you must drill and tap the coracoid process before the osteotomy is carried out. Otherwise, the small piece of coracoid may split during drilling, and anatomical reduction can be obtained only with extreme difficulty (Figs. 1-7 and 1-8).

The axillary artery is surrounded by the cords of the brachial plexus, which lie behind the pectoralis minor muscle. Abduction of the arm causes these neurovascular structures to become tight and brings them close to the tip of the coracoid and the operative site. Therefore, keep the arm adducted while working around the coracoid process (Fig. 1-9).[1]

Retract the coracoid (with its attached muscles) down and medially. Divide the fascia that fans out from the conjoint tendons of the coracobrachialis and the short head of the biceps on the lateral side of the coracobrachialis—the safe side of the muscle, since the musculocutaneous nerve enters the coracobrachialis on its medial side. Be careful as

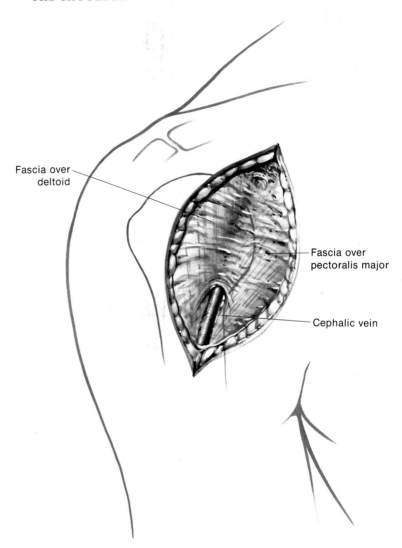

Fascia over
deltoid

Fascia over
pectoralis major

Cephalic vein

FIG. 1-6. Develop the groove between the fascia overlying the pectoralis major and the fascia overlying the deltoid. The cephalic vein will be of help in locating the groove.

you retract the coracoid with its attached muscles; overzealous downward retraction can cause a neurapraxia of the musculocutaneous nerve. If the coracoid process is left intact, the attached coracoid muscles protect the nerve from traction injury (Fig. 1-10).

Beneath the conjoint tendons of the coracobrachialis and the short head of biceps lie the transversely running fibers of the subscapularis muscle, which forms the only remaining anterior covering of the shoulder joint capsule (Fig. 1-11).[1] As the muscle crosses the glenoid cavity, a bursa separates it from the joint capsule; that bursa may communicate with the shoulder joint. In cases of multiple anterior dislocations, adhesions often exist between the muscle and the joint capsule, making the layer between the two difficult, if not impossible, to find.

Apply external rotation to the arm to stretch the subscapularis, bringing the muscle belly into the wound and making its superior and inferior borders easier to define. External rotation of the humerus also increases the distance between the subscapularis and the axillary nerve as it disappears below the lower border of the muscle (see Fig. 1-11).

The most identifiable landmarks on the inferior border of the subscapularis are a series of small transversely running vessels that often require ligation or cauterization. The vessels run as a triad: a small artery with its two surrounding venae comitantes, one above and one below the artery (Fig. 1-12).

Pass a blunt instrument between the capsule and the subscapularis from inferior to superior (see Fig. 1-12). Tag the muscle belly with stay

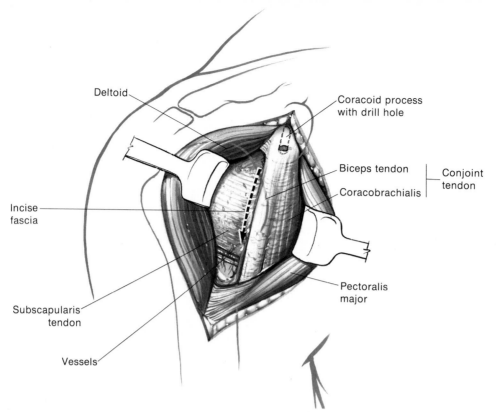

FIG. 1-7. Retract the pectoralis major medially and the deltoid laterally to expose the conjoint tendon of the short head of the biceps and coracobrachialis muscle. Drill the tip of the coracoid process before osteotomizing it. Incise the fascia over the subscapularis muscle on the lateral aspect of the conjoint tendon. Note the leash of vessels at the caudal end of the subscapularis muscle.

FIG. 1-8. Osteotomize the predrilled coracoid process. Retract the conjoint tendon laterally to give greater exposure to the subscapularis tendon.

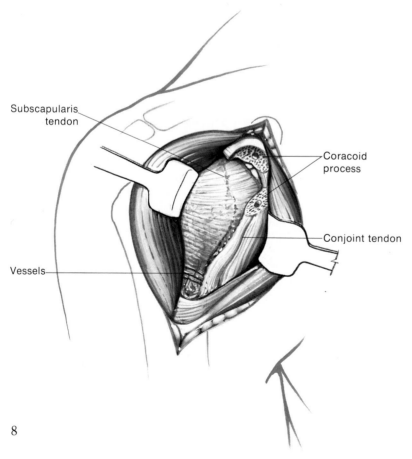

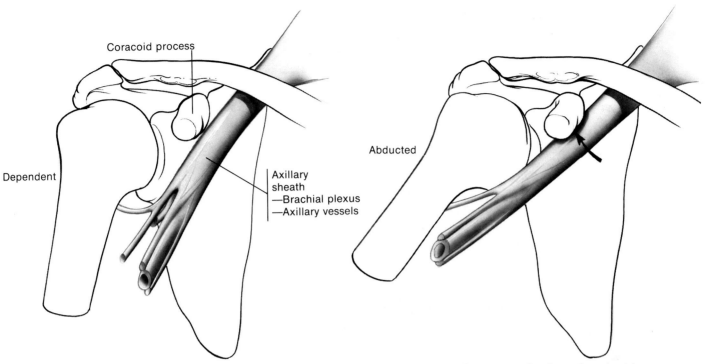

Coracoid process

Dependent

Abducted

Axillary
sheath
—Brachial plexus
—Axillary vessels

FIG. 1-9. Protect the axillary sheath by having the arm in the dependent position;
abduction of the arm will draw the sheath against the coracoid process.

FIG. 1-10. Vigorous retraction of the
conjoint tendon distally can injure the
musculocutaneous nerve, causing neurapraxia or avulsion.

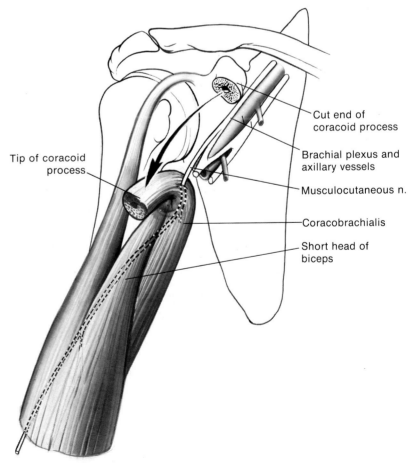

Tip of coracoid
process

Cut end of
coracoid process

Brachial plexus and
axillary vessels

Musculocutaneous n.

Coracobrachialis

Short head of
biceps

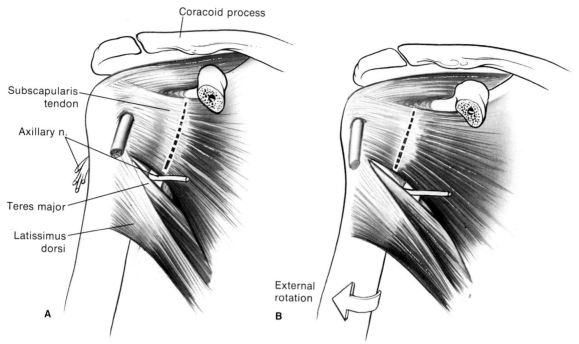

FIG. 1-11. (A) The subscapularis muscle lies in the deep part of the wound. It is to be incised perpendicular to its fibers, close to its tendon. The axillary nerve passes anteroposteriorly through the quadrangular space. **(B)** External rotation of the arm during incision into the subscapularis tendon will draw the point of incision away from the axillary nerve.

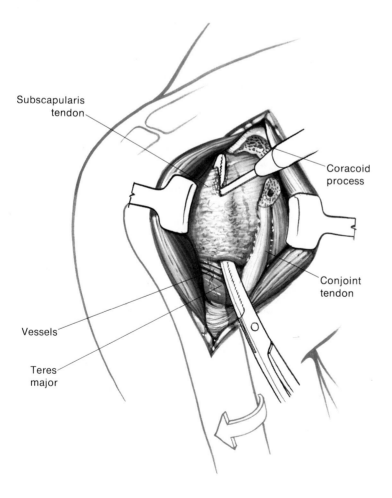

FIG. 1-12. Insert a Kelly clamp under the subscapularis muscle. A leash of vessels at the caudal end of the wound marks the lower border of the subscapularis.

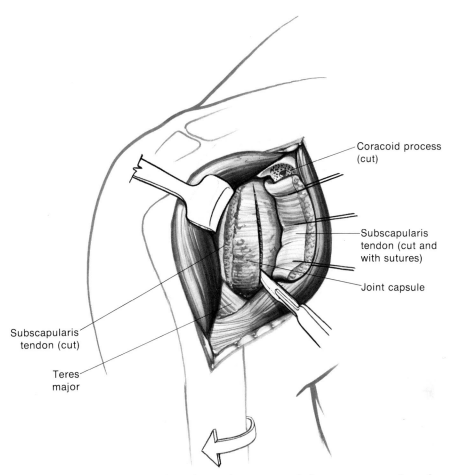

FIG. 1-13. Incise the end of the subscapularis. Tag and place stay sutures into the muscle to prevent it from retracting medially. Some of the subscapularis fibers insert directly into the joint capsule.

sutures to prevent it from disappearing medially when it is cut and to allow easy reattachment of the muscle to its new insertion onto the humerus. Then divide the subscapularis 1 inch from its insertion onto the lesser tuberosity of the humerus (Fig. 1-13). Note that some of its muscle fibers insert onto the joint capsule itself; frequently, the capsule may be opened inadvertently when the muscle is divided, since the two layers cannot always be defined.

Incise the capsule longitudinally to enter the joint wherever the selected repair must be performed. Each type of repair has its own specific location for incision (Fig. 1-14).

DANGERS

Nerves

The **musculocutaneous nerve** enters the body of the coracobrachialis about 5 cm to 8 cm distal to the muscle's origin at the coracoid process. Be-

cause the nerve enters the muscle from its medial side, all dissection must remain on the lateral side of the muscle. Take great care as you retract the muscle inferiorly, to avoid stretching the nerve and causing paralysis of the elbow flexors (see Fig. 1-10).

Vessels

The **cephalic vein** should be preserved, if possible, although ligation leads to few problems and prevents the slight danger of thromboembolism from traumatized vessels.

HOW TO ENLARGE THE APPROACH

Local Measures

The exposure can be enlarged in the following three ways:

1. Extend the skin incision superiorly by curving it laterally along the lower border of the clav-

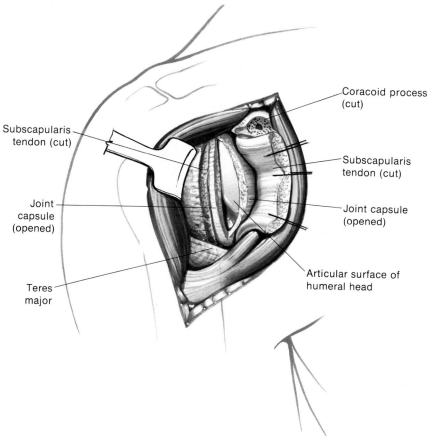

FIG. 1-14. Incise the joint capsule longitudinally to expose the humeral head and the glenoid cavity.

icle. Detach the deltoid from its origin on the outer surface of the clavicle for 2 cm to 4 cm to permit better lateral retraction of the muscle (Fig. 1-15). Unfortunately, because reattaching the deltoid may be difficult, this maneuver is not recommended for routine use. If further deltoid retraction is required, it may be best to detach part of the deltoid's insertion onto the humerus.

2. Lengthen the skin incision inferiorly along the deltopectoral groove to separate the pectoralis major from the deltoid further inferiorly and to improve the exposure without having to detach the deltoid origin.

3. Use a suitable retractor (like the Bankart skid) for the humeral head. A humeral head retractor is the key to excellent exposure of the inside of the glenoid fossa once the joint has been opened (Fig. 1-16).

Extensile Measures

PROXIMAL EXTENSION. To expose the brachial plexus and axillary artery and to gain control of arterial bleeding from the axillary artery, extend the skin incision superomedially, crossing the middle third of the clavicle. Next, dissect the middle third of the clavicle subperiosteally and osteotomize the bone, removing the middle third. Cut the subclavius muscle, which runs transversely under the clavicle. Retract the trapezius superiorly and the pectoralis major and pectoralis minor inferiorly to reveal the underlying axillary artery and the surrounding brachial plexus (Fig. 1-17). Take care not to damage the musculocutaneous nerve, the most superficial nerve in the brachial plexus.

DISTAL EXTENSION. The approach can be extended into an anterolateral approach to the humerus.

Extend the skin incision down the deltopectoral groove. Then curve it inferiorly, following the lateral border of the biceps. The deep dissection consists in moving the biceps brachii medially to reveal the underlying brachialis, which can then be split along the line of its fibers to provide access to the humerus. (For details of this approach, see Chapter 2, p. 48.)

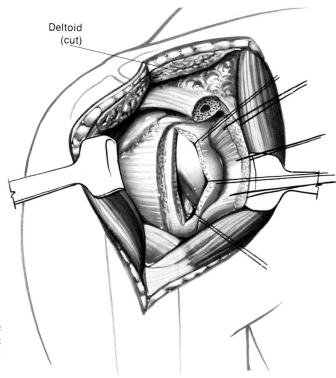

Deltoid
(cut)

FIG. 1-15. Remove the origins of the deltoid from the anterior portion of the clavicle to expose the joint further proximally. Identify the coracoacromial ligament.

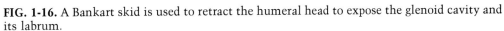

FIG. 1-16. A Bankart skid is used to retract the humeral head to expose the glenoid cavity and its labrum.

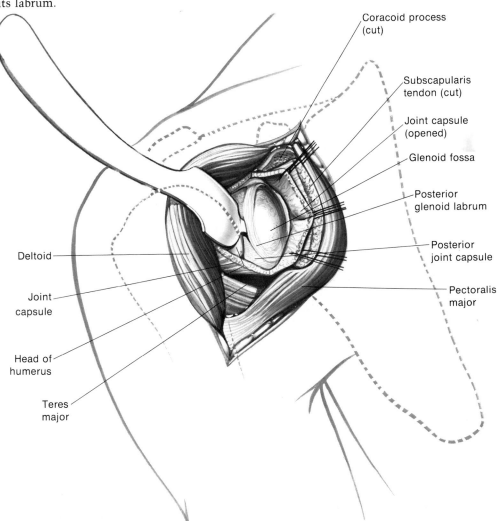

Coracoid process
(cut)

Subscapularis
tendon (cut)

Joint capsule
(opened)

Glenoid fossa

Posterior
glenoid labrum

Posterior
joint capsule

Pectoralis
major

Deltoid

Joint
capsule

Head of
humerus

Teres
major

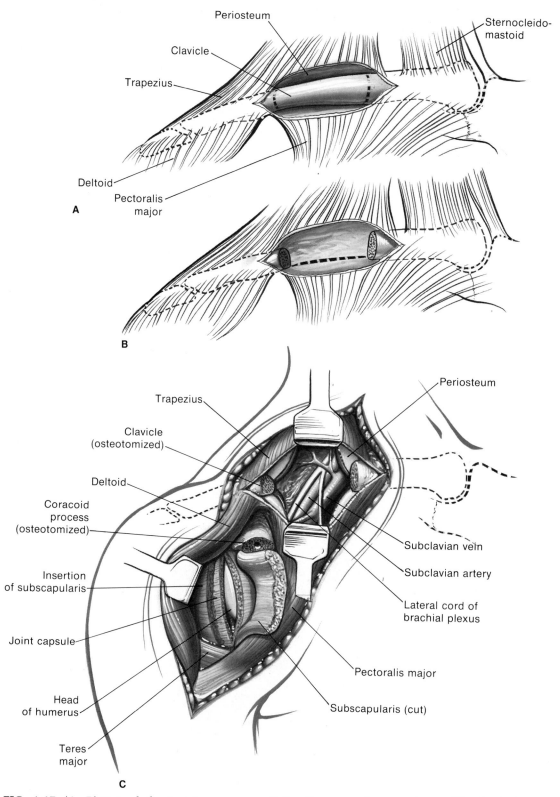

FIG. 1-17. (A, B) Extend the incision superomedially. Expose and resect the middle third of the clavicle subperiostally. **(C)** Expose the brachial plexus and axillary artery.

APPLIED SURGICAL ANATOMY OF THE ANTERIOR APPROACH

OVERVIEW

All approaches to the shoulder involve penetrating the two muscular coverings, or sleeves, that cover the joint. The outer sleeve is the deltoid muscle. The inner is the rotator cuff, which consists of four muscles: the supraspinatus, the infraspinatus, the teres minor, and the subscapularis (Fig. 1-18).

Anteriorly, access to the shoulder joint involves reflecting the outer sleeve laterally and incising the inner sleeve, specifically the subscapularis.

The deltoid, together with the pectoralis major and the latissimus dorsi (the two great muscles of the axillary fold), supplies most of the power required for shoulder movement. The muscles of the inner sleeve can all act as prime movers of the humerus, but their most important action is to control the humeral head within the glenoid cavity while the other muscles are carrying out major movements.

The supraspinatus has a key role as a prime mover of the humerus in initiating abduction. The teres minor and infraspinatus muscles are the only important external rotators of the shoulder. The pathology of the joint is nearly always associated with this inner group of muscles; their function is critical not only to the coordination of joint movement but also to the stability of the shoulder joint itself.

A third group of muscles intervenes between the two muscular sleeves when the joint is approached from the front. These muscles (the short head of the biceps, the coracobrachialis, and the pectoralis minor) require medial retraction for exposure of the inner sleeve. They are all attached to the coracoid process (see Fig. 1-18).

FIG. 1-18. Anatomy of the anterior portion of the shoulder.

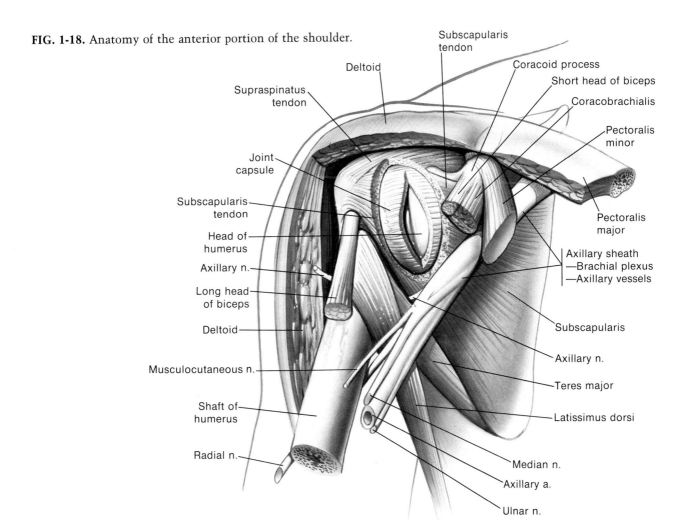

LANDMARKS AND INCISION

Landmarks

The *coracoid process of the scapula* is an accessible bony protuberance that lies at the upper end of the deltopectoral groove and is the landmark for incisions based on that groove. It is also a critical landmark for injections and arthroscopic examinations of the shoulder joint. Hook shaped, it is sometimes described as a crow's beak—as its name, corax implies. The tip of the coracoid projects forward, laterally, and inferiorly toward the glenoid cavity. Therefore, it is best palpated by posterior and medial pressure. Attached to it are the following five clinically important structures (Fig. 1-19):

Coracoacromial ligament. This tough fibrous ligament is triangular and connects the horizontal portion of the coracoid process to the tip of the acromion. It is one of the few ligaments that connects two parts of the same bone. The coracoid process, the acromion, and the coracoacromial ligament form the coracoacromial arch.

Conoid and trapezoid ligaments. These two coracoclavicular ligaments are extremely strong. The conoid ligament, which looks like an inverted cone, extends upward from the upper surface of the knuckle of the coracoid process to the undersurface of the clavicle. The trapezoid ligament runs from the upper surface of the coracoid process and extends superiorly and laterally to the trapezoid ridge on the undersurface of the clavicle. These two structures are the main

accessory ligaments of the acromioclavicular joint. They are extremely difficult to repair in cases of acromioclavicular dislocation and once torn are difficult to identify as individual structures.

Conjoint tendons of the coracobrachialis and biceps brachii (see p. 19)

Pectoralis minor (see p. 20)

Incision

Because a skin incision that runs down the deltopectoral groove cuts almost transversely across the cleavage lines of the skin, it often leaves a broad and ugly scar. An incision in the axilla runs with the cleavage line of the skin and leaves a much narrower scar. That scar is almost invisible, because it is hidden in the axillary fold and covered by hair.

SUPERFICIAL SURGICAL DISSECTION

Three major structures are involved in the superficial surgical dissection of the anterior approach to the shoulder joint: the deltoid muscle laterally; the pectoralis major medially; and the cephalic vein, which lies between them in the deltopectoral groove (Fig. 1-20).

Deltoid

The anterior fibers of the deltoid run parallel to each other, without fibrous septa between fibers. Because sutures placed in this kind of muscle fiber tend to tear out, it is difficult to reattach the del-

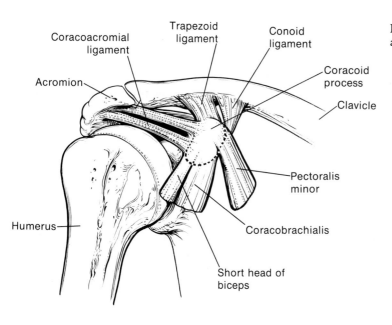

Coracoacromial ligament

Trapezoid ligament

Conoid ligament

Acromion

Coracoid process

Clavicle

Pectoralis minor

Coracobrachialis

Humerus

Short head of biceps

FIG. 1-19. Five clinically important structures are attached to the coracoid process.

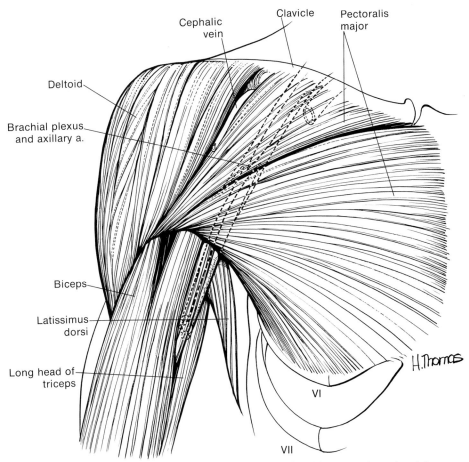

Cephalic vein

Clavicle

Pectoralis major

Deltoid

Brachial plexus and axillary a.

Biceps

Latissimus dorsi

Long head of triceps

VI

VII

H.Thomas

FIG. 1-20. The superficial anatomy of the anterior shoulder, revealing the deltopectoral groove and the neurovascular bundle.

toid to the clavicle. Sutures must be placed through the full thickness of the muscle, including its fascial coverings, to effect a strong reattachment. The attachment should be protected from active stress for 4 weeks to allow for adequate healing.

The anterior portion of the deltoid can be denervated only if the entire anterior part of the muscle is stripped and retracted vigorously in a lateral direction (Fig. 1-21).

Pectoralis Major

The two nerve supplies of the pectoralis major allow the muscle to be split without the loss of nerve supply to either part, making possible muscle transfers like the Clark procedure, in which the distal part of the muscle is separated from the proximal part and inserted into the biceps tendon in the arm (see Fig. 1-21).[10]

Cephalic Vein

The cephalic vein drains into the axillary vein after passing through the clavipectoral fascia. On occasion, it may be absent. Few complications result from its ligation (see Fig. 1-20).

DEEP SURGICAL DISSECTION

The coracobrachialis and the short head of the biceps brachii share a common origin from the tip of the coracoid process. They also share a common nerve supply, the musculocutaneous nerve. They form an intermediate layer during the approach (Fig. 1-22).

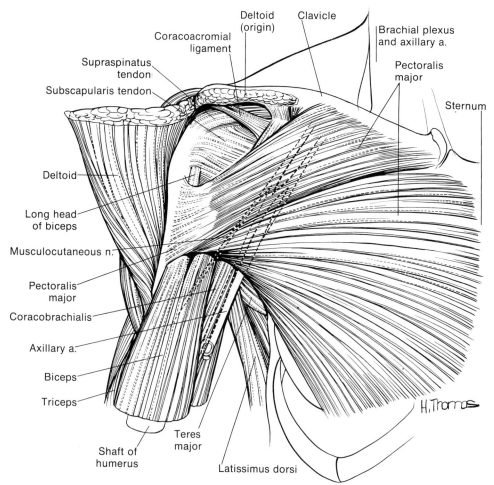

FIG 1-21. The anterior portion of the deltoid has been resected from its origin, revealing the insertion of the pectoralis major muscle and the subscapularis tendon, supraspinatus tendon, and coracoacromial ligament.

Coracobrachialis

The coracobrachialis is largely vestigial and has little function. Extremely variable in size, it is the arm's counterpart of the adductors of the thigh.

The coracobrachialis used to have three heads of origin. The musculocutaneous nerve passes between two of the original heads, now fused during development. Its course is one of the few times a nerve appears to pass through a muscle. When a nerve does this, it is always passing between two heads of origin (see Fig. 1-22).

Biceps Brachii

The tendon of the long head of the biceps is an anatomical curiosity; it is one of only two tendons to pass through a synovial cavity. The joint capsule of the shoulder is incomplete inferiorly, so the tendon can escape under the transverse ligament. From there it runs in the bicipital groove of the

humerus. It is easy to palpate the tendon in the groove as long as the arm is externally rotated (see Fig. 1-24). The biceps tendon is a common site of inflammatory changes, partly because it is capable of tremendous excursion, moving some 6 cm between full abduction and full adduction of the shoulder. This continual movement may produce attrition between the tendon and the bicipital groove. The tendon may also rupture, producing a characteristic change in the contour of the muscle.

The biceps can slip medially out of the bicipital groove. This dislocation is usually painful,[11] although dislocation is sometimes found during postmortems of people who have had no known shoulder symptomatology.[12]

Considerable variability exists in the depth of the bicipital groove and in the angle that its medial wall makes with its floor.[13] Shallow grooves with

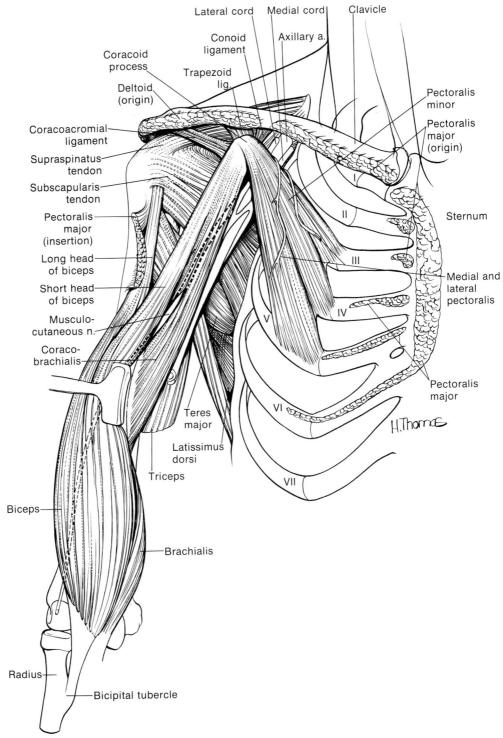

FIG. 1-22. The pectoralis major and deltoid muscles have been completely removed, revealing the two heads of the biceps tendon, the rotator cuff, the coracoacromial ligament, and the neurovascular bundle.

flat medial walls may be predisposed to such tendon dislocation. Nevertheless, the transverse humeral ligament (retinaculum), the chief stabilizer for the tendon, must be ruptured before the tendon can be displaced.

Pectoralis Minor

The only surgical importance of the pectoralis minor muscle lies in its neurovascular relations. The second part of the axillary artery and the cords of the brachial plexus lie directly behind the muscle and below the coracoid process (see Fig. 1-22).

Subscapularis

The deep layer of the dissection is formed by the subscapularis muscle, which covers the shoulder joint capsule.

The subscapularis, the anterior portion of the rotator cuff, inserts partly into the capsule of the joint. The muscle tendon undergoes degeneration in the same way as do other muscles of the rotator cuff, but to a lesser extent. The problem is rarely severe or symptomatic because there are other internal rotators of the shoulder, and loss of subscapularis action is not functionally disabling. The subscapularis may be stretched in cases of anterior dislocations of the shoulder or may be contracted as a result of previous surgery.[13]

The subscapularis limits external rotation, helping to prevent anterior dislocations; it may also physically block anterior dislocation because of its size and its position in front of the shoulder joint. Because the two subscapular nerves enter the muscle medially, incising it 2.5 cm from its insertion does not denervate the muscle (Fig. 1-23).

Superiorly, the muscle is intimately connected to the supraspinatus. The plane of cleavage between the two muscles, a true internervous plane between the suprascapular and subscapular nerves, may be difficult to define, especially near the insertions of the muscles. The tendon of the long head of the biceps corresponds to the interval between the muscles and can be used as a surgical guideline to that interval.

Shoulder Joint Capsule

The shoulder joint has an enormous range of motion. The capsule is loose and redundant, particularly inferiorly and anteriorly. The area of the fibrous capsule itself is approximately twice the surface area of the humeral head (see Fig. 1-23). Anteriorly, the capsule is attached to the scapula via the border of the glenoid labrum and the bone next to it. The anterior part of the capsule usually has a small gap that allows the synovial lining of the joint to communicate with the bursa underlying the subscapularis.[14,15] This bursa extends across the front of the neck of the scapula toward the coracoid process (Fig. 1-24; see Fig. 1-36).

Posteriorly and inferiorly, the capsule is attached to the border of the labrum. A second gap may exist here to allow communication between the synovial lining of the joint and the infraspinatus bursa.

The fibrous capsule inserts into the humerus around the articular margins of the neck, except inferiorly where the insertion is a centimeter below the articular margin. The capsule bridges the gap across the bicipital groove, forming a structure known as the transverse ligament. The long head of the biceps enters the joint beneath this ligament (see Fig. 1-24).

The shoulder joint capsule receives reinforcement from all four muscles of the rotator cuff. Further reinforcement is provided by the three glenohumeral ligaments, which appear as thickenings in the capsule. These ligaments are extremely difficult to identify during surgery and are of no clinical relevance.

Synovial Lining of the Shoulder Joint

The synovial membrane, which is attached around the glenoid labrum, lines the capsule of the joint. The membrane usually communicates with the subscapularis bursa and, occasionally, with the infraspinatus bursa (see Figs. 1-24 and 1-36). It envelopes the tendon of the long head of the biceps within the shoulder joint. The synovium forms a tubular sleeve that permits the tendon to glide back and forth during abduction and adduction of the arm. Therefore, the tendon is anatomically intracapsular, but extrasynovial (Fig. 1-25; see Fig. 1-36).

Glenoid Labrum

The glenoid labrum is a triangular fibrocartilaginous structure that rings the glenoid cavity (see Fig. 1-25). The joint capsule attaches to it superiorly, inferiorly, and posteriorly. Anteriorly, the attachment depends on the presence or absence of the synovial recess running across the scapular neck (subscapularis bursa) (see Fig. 1-36); the presence of the synovial recess leaves a gap in the attachment of the glenoid to the scapula (see Fig. 1-24).

It is the detachment of the glenoid labrum anteriorly that creates the Bankart lesion in cases of recurrent anterior dislocation of the shoulder (Fig. 1-26).

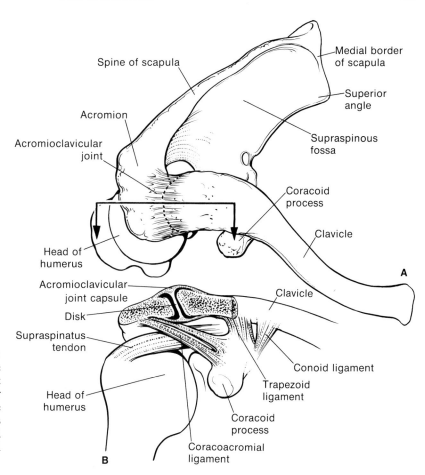

FIG. 1-41. **(A)** Superior view of the shoulder joint, revealing the bone structure and acromioclavicular joint capsule. **(B)** Cross section of anterior view of the shoulder, revealing the acromioclavicular joint and meniscus as well as the supraspinatus tendon and its relationship to the coracoacromial ligament.

palpate the joint by pushing medially against the thickness at the end of the clavicle.

The joint contains a fibrocartilaginous meniscus, which is usually incomplete; the meniscus may be displaced during traumatic subluxation of the joint (Fig. 1-41*B*).

The major surgical importance of the joint occurs in cases of acromioclavicular dislocation or acromioclavicular arthritis. The major accessory ligaments of the joint, from the coracoid process to the undersurface of the clavicle, are some distance from it; they cannot be repaired, but they can, and

should, be replaced if the joint is to be rendered stable.

The joint is easily exposed by way of a superior approach because it is essentially subcutaneous. The insertions of the trapezius and the deltoid to the superior surface of the clavicle are confluent, and the two muscles are easily separated by subperiosteal dissection (Fig. 1-42). In cases of acromioclavicular separation, however, it may be necessary to detach some of the deltoid from the clavicle to expose the coracoid, coracoclavicular, and acromioclavicular ligaments (Fig. 1-41).

POSTERIOR APPROACH

The posterior approach offers access to the posterior and inferior aspects of the shoulder joint.[24] It is rarely needed. Its uses include the following:

1. Repairs in cases of recurrent posterior dislocation or subluxation of the shoulder[25,26]
2. Glenoid osteotomy[27]

3. Biopsy and excision of tumors
4. Removal of loose bodies in the posterior recess of the shoulder
5. Drainage of sepsis (the approach allows dependent drainage with the patient in the normal position in bed)

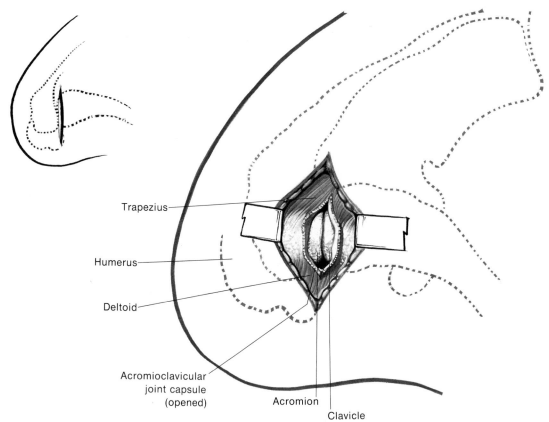

FIG. 1-42. Superior approach to the acromioclavicular joint.

POSITION OF PATIENT

Place the patient in a lateral position on the edge of the operating table, with his affected side uppermost; drape the patient to allow independent movement of his arm (Fig. 1-43). Stand behind the patient. Take care that the patient's ear is not accidentally folded under his head.

LANDMARKS AND INCISION

Landmarks

The *acromion* and the *spine of the scapula* form one continuous arch. The spine of the scapula extends obliquely across the upper four fifths of the dorsum of the scapula and ends in a flat, smooth triangle at the medial border of the scapula. It is easy to palpate.

Incision

Make a linear incision along the entire length of the scapular spine, extending to the posterior corner of the acromion (Fig. 1-44).

INTERNERVOUS PLANE

The internervous plane lies between the *teres minor*, supplied by the axillary nerve, and the *infraspinatus*, supplied by the suprascapular nerve (Fig. 1-45).

SUPERFICIAL SURGICAL DISSECTION

Identify the origin of the deltoid on the scapular spine and detach the muscle from this origin. The plane between the deltoid and the underlying infraspinatus may be difficult to find, mainly because there is a tendency to look for it too close to bone and to end up stripping the infraspinatus off the scapula. The plane is easier to locate at the lateral end of the incision. Once it has been found, it is not difficult to develop if you retract the deltoid inferiorly and expose the infraspinatus (Fig. 1-46). Note that the plane is also an internervous plane, since the deltoid is supplied by the axillary nerve and the infraspinatus by the suprascapular nerve.

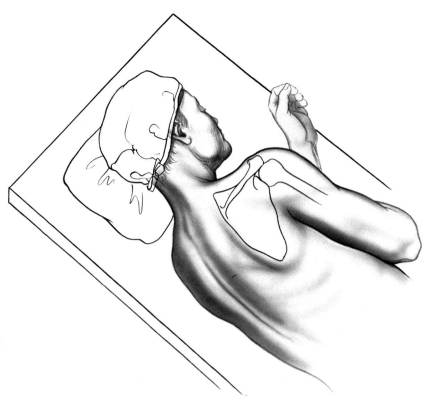

FIG. 1-43. Position of the patient on the operating table for the posterior approach to the shoulder. Drape the involved arm to allow for independent motion.

FIG. 1-44. Make a linear incision over the entire length of the scapular spine, extending to the posterior corner of the acromion. You may choose to curve the medial end of the incision distally to enhance the exposure.

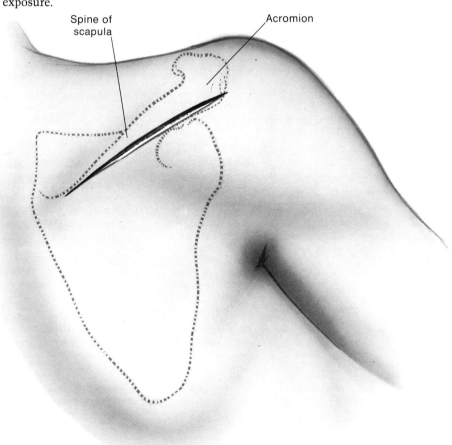

Spine of
scapula

Acromion

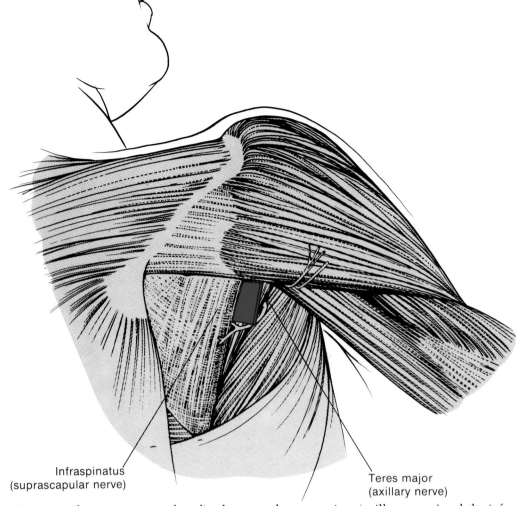

Infraspinatus
(suprascapular nerve)

Teres major
(axillary nerve)

FIG. 1-45. The internervous plane lies between the teres minor (axillary nerve) and the infraspinatus (suprascapular nerve).

DEEP SURGICAL DISSECTION

Identify the internervous plane between the infraspinatus and the teres minor and develop it by blunt dissection, using your finger. This important plane is difficult to define (Fig. 1-47). Retract the infraspinatus superiorly and the teres minor inferiorly to reach the posterior regions of the glenoid cavity and the neck of the scapula (Fig. 1-48). The posteroinferior corner of the shoulder joint capsule is now exposed. To explore the joint, incise it longitudinally, close to the edge of the scapula (Figs. 1-49 and 1-50).

DANGERS

Nerves

The **axillary nerve** runs through the quadrangular space beneath the teres minor. Because a dissection carried out inferior to the teres minor can damage the axillary nerve, it is critical to identify the muscular interval between the infraspinatus and the teres minor and to stay within that interval.

The **suprascapular nerve** passes around the base of the spine of the scapula as it runs from the supraspinous fossa to the infraspinous fossa. It is the nerve supply for both supraspinatus and infraspinatus. The infraspinatus must not be forcefully retracted too far medially during the approach lest a neurapraxia result from stretching the nerve around the unyielding lateral edge of the scapular spine (see Fig. 1-54).

Vessels

The **posterior circumflex humeral artery** runs with the axillary nerve in the quadrangular space beneath the inferior border of the teres minor. Damage to this artery leads to hemorrhaging that is difficult to control. You can avoid the danger by staying in the correct intermuscular plane (see Fig. 1-53).

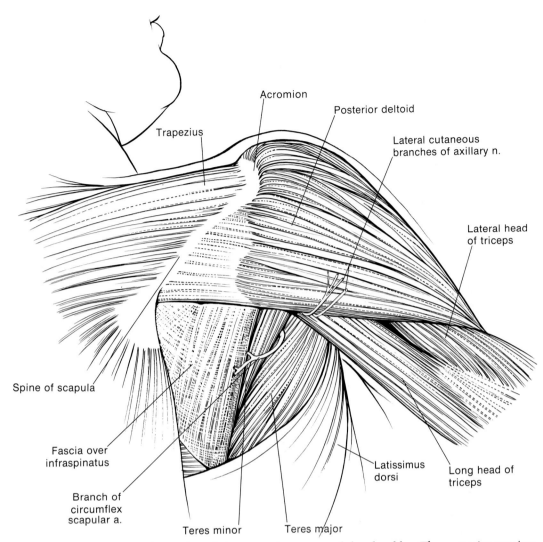

FIG. 1-52. The superficial muscles of the posterior aspect of the shoulder. The posterior portion of the deltoid as it takes origin from the spine of the scapula is aponeurotic, and the plane between it and the underlying infraspinatus is difficult to identify.

from above; part of the deltoid originates from its inferior border (see Fig. 1-52).

Incision

Because the transverse skin incision runs across the lines of cleavage of the skin, the resultant scar is usually broad. A vertical incision at the lateral end of the scapular spine is more cosmetic but gives poor exposure of the joint.

SUPERFICIAL SURGICAL DISSECTION

In the posterior approach, only those fibers of the deltoid that arise from the spine of the scapula are detached. Because the fibers are straight and blend

intimately with the periosteum of the scapula, the muscle can be removed subperiosteally. During closure, the good, tough tissue that remains attached to the muscle provides an excellent anchor for sutures, in contrast to the anterior and lateral portions of the muscle (see p. 30). However, you may need to put drill holes through the spine to anchor the muscular sutures.

DEEP SURGICAL DISSECTION

The deep dissection in this approach lies between the infraspinatus and the teres minor (see Fig. 1-53).

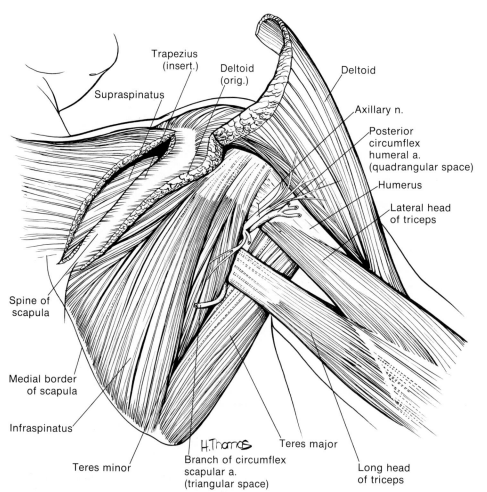

FIG. 1-53. The posterior portion of the deltoid is detached from the spine of the scapula, revealing the infraspinatus, teres minor, and teres major muscles, as well as the long and lateral heads of the triceps muscle. The boundaries of the quadrangular space are, superiorly, the lower border of the teres minor; laterally, the surgical neck of the humerus; medially, the long head of the triceps; and, anteriorly, the upper border of the teres major. Through this space run the axillary nerve and the posterior circumflex humeral artery.

Infraspinatus. *Origin.* Medial three fourths of infraspinous fossa of scapula. *Insertion.* Central facet on greater tuberosity of humerus. *Action.* Lateral rotator of humerus. *Nerve supply.* Suprascapular nerve.

Teres Minor. *Origin.* Axillary border of scapula. *Insertion.* Lowest facet on greater tuberosity of humerus. *Action.* Lateral rotator of humerus. *Nerve supply.* Axillary nerve.

Infraspinatus

The fibers of the infraspinatus are multipennate; numerous fibrous intramuscular septa give attachment to them.

The infraspinatus forms its tendon just before crossing the back of the shoulder joint; a small bursa lies between the muscle and the posterior aspect of the scapular neck to help the tendon glide freely over the bone. The muscle also inserts into the capsule of the shoulder joint, mechanically increasing the capsule's strength (Fig. 1-54).

Teres Minor

The teres minor runs side by side with the infraspinatus. Its fibers run parallel with one another, in contrast to the multipennate fibers of the infraspinatus, a difference that may help you pick up the interval between the two muscles.

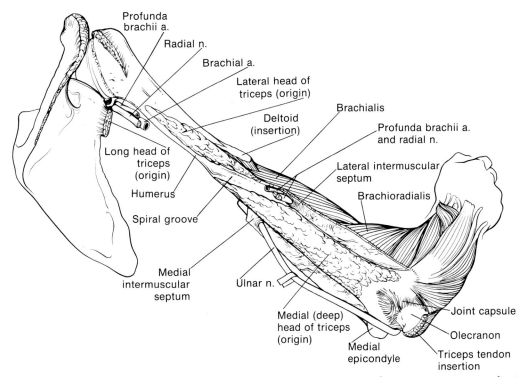

Profunda brachii a.

Radial n.

Brachial a.

Lateral head of triceps (origin)

Deltoid (insertion)

Brachialis

Profunda brachii a. and radial n.

Lateral intermuscular septum

Brachioradialis

Long head of triceps (origin)

Humerus

Spiral groove

Medial intermuscular septum

Ulnar n.

Medial (deep) head of triceps (origin)

Medial epicondyle

Joint capsule

Olecranon

Triceps tendon insertion

FIG. 2-37. The entire triceps muscle has been removed, uncovering the entire posterior surface of the humerus. The medial and lateral intermuscular septa and the nerves that penetrate them are seen.

FIG. 2-38. The lateral aspect of the humerus, with the overlying superficial cutaneous nerves.

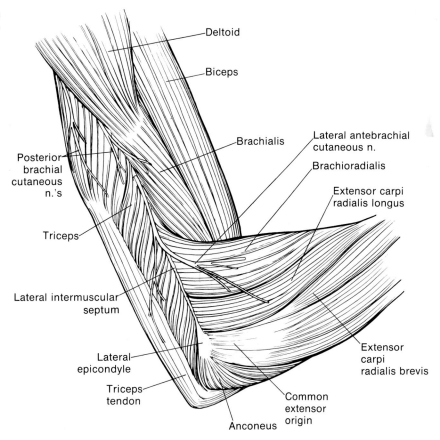

Deltoid

Biceps

Brachialis

Lateral antebrachial cutaneous n.

Brachioradialis

Extensor carpi radialis longus

Posterior brachial cutaneous n.'s

Triceps

Lateral intermuscular septum

Lateral epicondyle

Triceps tendon

Anconeus

Common extensor origin

Extensor carpi radialis brevis

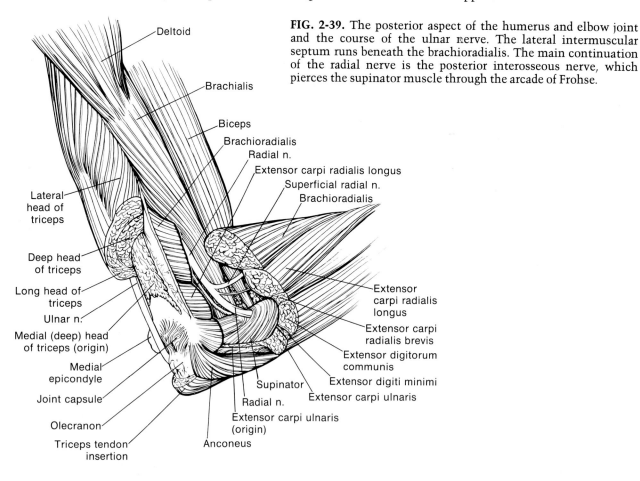

FIG. 2-39. The posterior aspect of the humerus and elbow joint and the course of the ulnar nerve. The lateral intermuscular septum runs beneath the brachioradialis. The main continuation of the radial nerve is the posterior interosseous nerve, which pierces the supinator muscle through the arcade of Frohse.

Deltoid

Brachialis

Biceps

Brachioradialis

Radial n.

Extensor carpi radialis longus

Superficial radial n.

Brachioradialis

Lateral head of triceps

Deep head of triceps

Long head of triceps

Ulnar n.

Medial (deep) head of triceps (origin)

Medial epicondyle

Joint capsule

Olecranon

Triceps tendon insertion

Anconeus

Supinator

Radial n.

Extensor carpi ulnaris (origin)

Extensor carpi ulnaris

Extensor digiti minimi

Extensor digitorum communis

Extensor carpi radialis brevis

Extensor carpi radialis longus

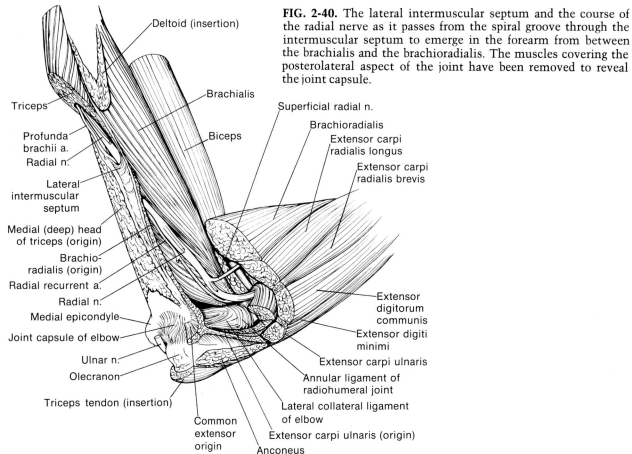

FIG. 2-40. The lateral intermuscular septum and the course of the radial nerve as it passes from the spiral groove through the intermuscular septum to emerge in the forearm from between the brachialis and the brachioradialis. The muscles covering the posterolateral aspect of the joint have been removed to reveal the joint capsule.

Deltoid (insertion)

Brachialis

Biceps

Superficial radial n.

Brachioradialis

Extensor carpi radialis longus

Extensor carpi radialis brevis

Triceps

Profunda brachii a.

Radial n.

Lateral intermuscular septum

Medial (deep) head of triceps (origin)

Brachio-radialis (origin)

Radial recurrent a.

Radial n.

Medial epicondyle

Joint capsule of elbow

Ulnar n.

Olecranon

Triceps tendon (insertion)

Common extensor origin

Extensor digitorum communis

Extensor digiti minimi

Extensor carpi ulnaris

Annular ligament of radiohumeral joint

Lateral collateral ligament of elbow

Extensor carpi ulnaris (origin)

Anconeus

FIG. 2-41. The muscles have been completely removed, showing the origins of the musculature of the posterior humerus.

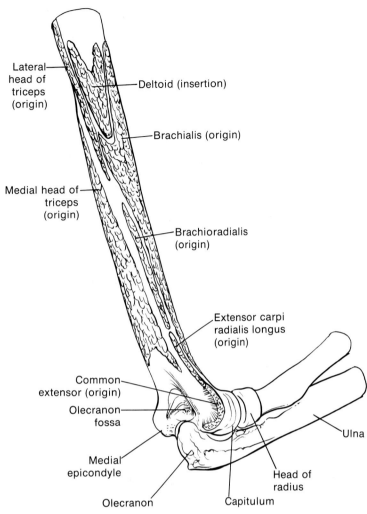

Lateral head of triceps (origin)

Deltoid (insertion)

Brachialis (origin)

Medial head of triceps (origin)

Brachioradialis (origin)

Extensor carpi radialis longus (origin)

Common extensor (origin)

Olecranon fossa

Ulna

Medial epicondyle

Head of radius

Olecranon

Capitulum

REFERENCES

1. HENRY AK: Extensile Exposure, 2nd ed. Edinburgh, E&S Livingston, 1966
2. HENRY AK: Exposure of the humerus and femoral shaft. Br J Surg 12:84, 1924–1925
3. THOMPSON JE: Anatomical methods of approach in operating on the long bones of the extremities. Ann Surg 68:309, 1918
4. BOYD HB, MCLEOD AC JR: Tennis elbow. J Bone Joint Surg (Am) 55:1183, 1973
5. LAST RJ: Anatomy Regional and Applied, 6th ed. Edinburgh, Churchill Livingstone, 1978
6. STRUTHERS J: On a peculiarity of the humerus and humeral artery. Monthly J Med Sci 8:264, 1948
7. SUTHERLAND S: Nerves and Nerve Injuries. Baltimore, Williams & Wilkins, 1968

3

The Elbow

The elbow is a hinged joint, supported by strong collateral ligaments. The key neurovascular structures running down the arm pass anterior and posterior to the joint. The medial and lateral approaches, therefore, avoid the obvious neurovascular dangers but give limited access to the joint because of its bony configuration. Anterior and posterior approaches give better access to the joint but may endanger the key neurovascular structures.

Of the five approaches described, the *posterior approach* gives the best possible exposure to all the joint's surfaces and is the one most often used for the internal fixation of complex fractures of the elbow joint. The *medial approach* gives good access to the medial side of the joint, but for best exposure it does require an osteotomy of the medial epicondyle. However, this osteotomy does not involve any part of the articular surface. Although the approach is extensile to the distal humerus, it is most useful in dealing with local pathologies of the medial side of the joint. The *anterolateral approach* exposes the lateral side of the joint; in addition, it can be extended both proximally and distally to expose both humerus and radius from the shoulder to the wrist. The *anterior approach* to the cubital fossa is an approach designed primarily for exploration of the critical neurovascular structures that pass in front of the elbow joint. The *posterolateral approach* to the radial head is an approach designed exclusively for surgery to that structure.

The applied anatomy of the elbow is discussed in a single section after the approaches, mainly because the keys to the surgical anatomy are the neurovascular bundles that pass across the elbow joint; their positions are important in all of the approaches. Separate subsections are included in the anatomy section for specific anatomy that applies to each particular approach.

POSTERIOR APPROACH

The posterior approach gives the best possible view of the bones that comprise the elbow joint.[1] A safe, reliable approach, it does, however, have one major drawback: It usually requires an osteotomy of the olecranon on its articular surface, creating another "fracture," which must be internally fixed. Its uses include the following:

1. Open reduction and internal fixation of fractures of the distal humerus[2,3]
2. Removal of loose bodies within the elbow joint
3. Treatment of nonunions of the distal humerus

Extension contractures of the elbow can be treated by using part of this approach to lengthen the triceps, which does not require an olecranon osteotomy.

POSITION OF PATIENT

Place the patient supine on the operating table, with his arm across his chest. Exsanguinate the limb by elevating it for 3 to 5 minutes, and then apply a tourniquet (Fig. 3-1).

LANDMARKS AND INCISION

Landmark

Palpate the large, bony *olecranon process* at the upper end of the ulna. It is conical and has a relatively sharp apex.

Incision

Make a longitudinal incision on the posterior aspect of the elbow. Begin 5 cm above the olecranon in the midline of the posterior aspect of the arm. Just above the tip of the olecranon, curve the incision laterally so that it runs down the lateral side of the process. To complete the incision, curve it medially again so that it overlies the middle of the subcutaneous surface of the ulna. Running the incision around the tip of the olecranon moves the suture line away from devices that are used to fix the olecranon osteotomy and away from the weight-bearing tip of the elbow (Fig. 3-2).

INTERNERVOUS PLANE

There is no true internervous plane, since the approach involves little more than detaching the extensor mechanism of the elbow. The nerve supply of the triceps (radial nerve) enters the muscle well proximal to dissection up the arm.

SUPERFICIAL SURGICAL DISSECTION

Incise the deep fascia in the midline. Palpate the ulnar nerve as it lies in the bony groove on the back of the medial epicondyle, and incise the fascia overlying the nerve to expose it. Fully dissect out the ulnar nerve and pass tapes around it so that you can identify it at all times (Fig. 3-3).

If you are going to use a screw to fix the olecranon osteotomy, predrill and tap the olecranon *before* you perform the osteotomy. Score the bone

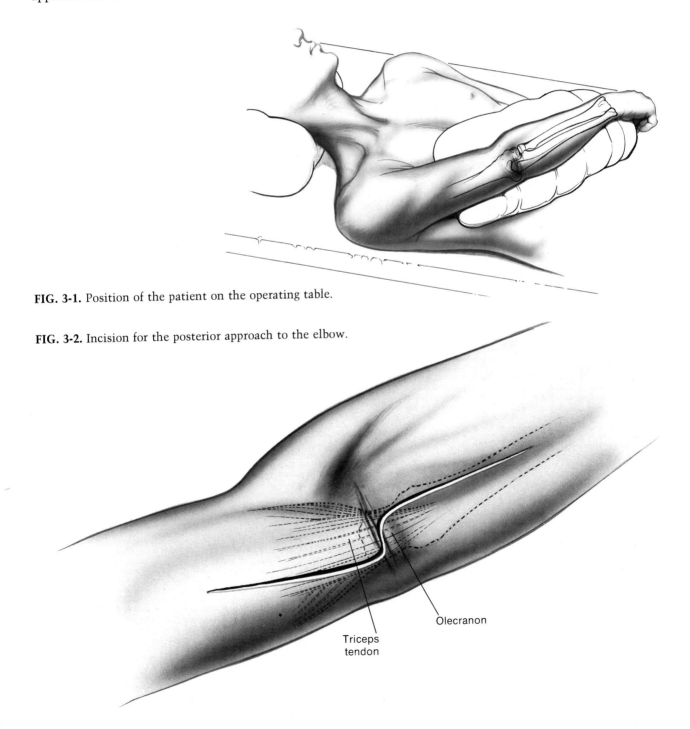

FIG. 3-1. Position of the patient on the operating table.

FIG. 3-2. Incision for the posterior approach to the elbow.

Olecranon

Triceps tendon

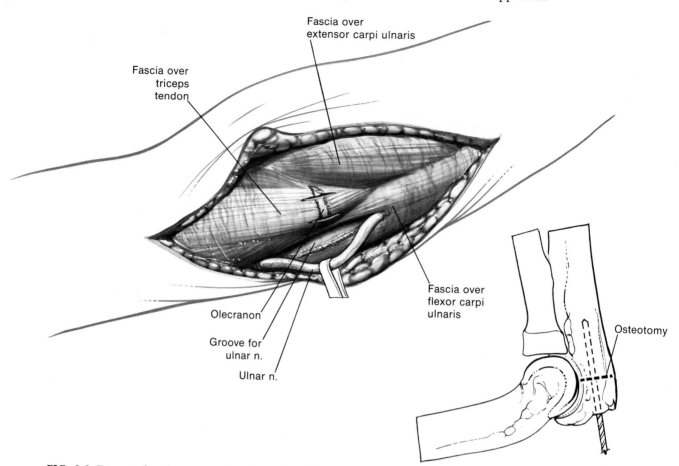

FIG. 3-3. Dissect the ulnar nerve from its bed and hold it free with tape. Predrill the olecranon before you perform an osteotomy for easy reattachment.

longitudinally with an osteotome so that you can correctly align the pieces when you repair the osteotomy (Fig. 3-3 *inset*).

Make a transverse osteotomy of the olecranon about 2 cm from its tip, using an oscillating saw.

DEEP SURGICAL DISSECTION

Strip the soft tissue attachments off the medial and lateral sides of the osteotomized portion of the olecranon and retract it proximally, elevating the triceps from the back of the humerus (Fig. 3-4 and *inset*). The posterior aspect of the distal end of the humerus is directly underneath; subperiosteal dissection around the medial and lateral borders of the bone allows you to expose all surfaces of the distal fourth of the humerus (Fig. 3-5 and *inset*). Note that you will will seldom need the full exposure. All the soft tissue attachments to bone that can be preserved should be, particularly in reductions of fractures. Stripping excessive soft tissue attachments off the bone leaves the bone's fragments avascular and jeopardizes its healing.

Be careful not to extend the dissection proximally above the distal fourth of the humerus, since the radial nerve, which passes from the posterior to the anterior compartment of the arm through the lateral intermuscular septum, may be damaged. Flex the elbow to relax the anterior structures if you need to elevate them off the front of the humerus (see Figs. 2-35 and 2-36).

The ulnar nerve must be kept clear of the operative field during all stages of the dissection. Some surgeons advise routine anterior transposition of the nerve during closure.

DANGERS

Nerves

The **ulnar nerve** is in no danger as long as it is identified early and protected and you avoid excessive traction on it.

The **median nerve** lies anterior to the distal humerus. It may be endangered if the stripping of the anterior structures off the distal humerus is not carried out strictly in a subperiosteal plane (see Fig. 3-5 *inset*).

The **radial nerve** is in danger if the dissection ventures farther proximally than the distal third of the humerus, one handbreadth above the lateral epicondyle (see Fig. 2-35).

Vessels

The **brachial artery** lies with the median nerve in front of the elbow. It should be afforded the same protection as the nerve (see Fig. 3-5 *inset*).

SPECIAL POINTS

Great care must be taken to realign the olecranon correctly during closure. Alignment following fractures is easy, since the uneven ends of the bone usually fit snugly, like a jigsaw puzzle. However, osteotomies result in flat surfaces and can make accurate reattachment difficult (see Fig. 3-3 and *inset*).

HOW TO ENLARGE THE APPROACH

Extensile Measures

PROXIMAL EXTENSION. The approach cannot be extended more proximally than the distal third of the humerus because of the danger to the radial nerve (see Fig. 2-35).

DISTAL EXTENSION. The incision can be continued along the subcutaneous border of the ulna, exposing the entire length of that bone (see pp. 124–127).

FIG. 3-4. Perform a transverse osteotomy of the olecranon and retract it proximally, with the triceps muscle attached. Strip a portion of the joint capsule with an osteotome.

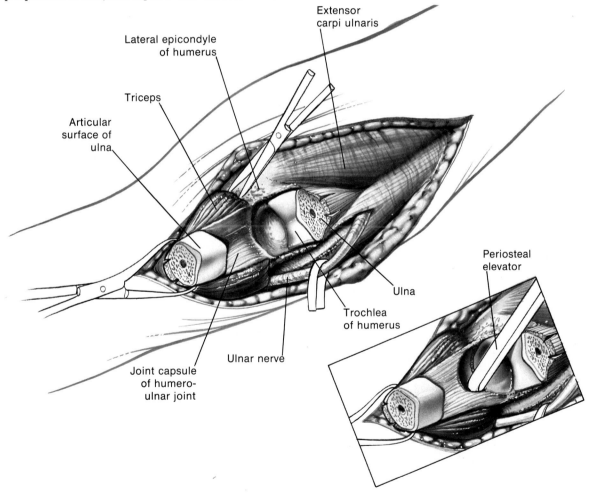

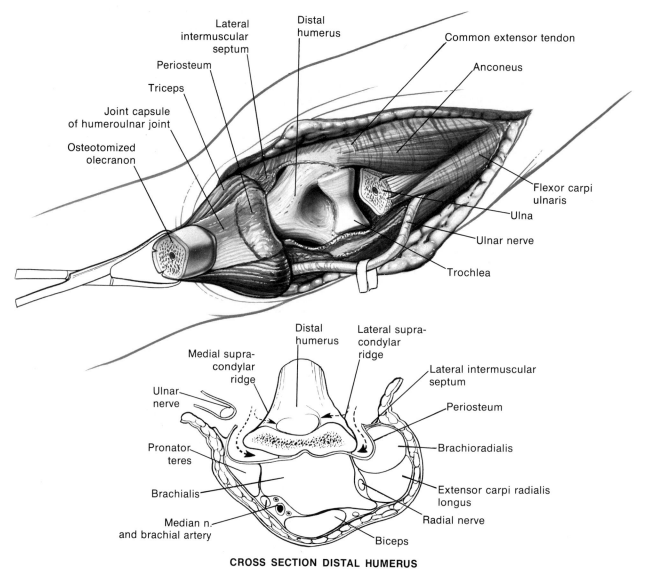

CROSS SECTION DISTAL HUMERUS

FIG. 3-5. Dissect around the medial and lateral borders of the bone to expose all the surfaces of the distal fourth of the humerus.

MEDIAL APPROACH

The medial approach gives good exposure of the medial compartment of the joint.[4,5] It can also be enlarged to expose the anterior surface of the distal fourth of the humerus. The ulnar nerve, which runs across the operative field, and the median nerve and brachial artery may be at risk in this exposure. The uses of the medial approach include the following:

1. Removal of loose bodies
2. Open reduction and internal fixation of fractures of the coronoid process of the ulna
3. Open reduction and internal fixation of fractures of the medial humeral condyle and epicondyle

The medial approach gives poor access to the lateral side of the joint and should not be used for routine exploration of the elbow. However, you may dislocate the joint during the procedure to gain access to the lateral side of the joint, if necessary.

POSITION OF PATIENT

Place the patient supine on the operating table, with his arm supported on an arm board or table. Abduct the arm and fully externally rotate the shoulder so that the medial epicondyle of the humerus faces anteriorly. Flex the elbow 90° (Fig. 3-6).

Exsanguinate the limb either by elevating it for 5 minutes or by applying a soft rubber bandage. Next, inflate a tourniquet.

LANDMARKS AND INCISION

Landmarks

Palpate the *medial epicondyle of the humerus,* the large subcutaneous bony mass that stands out on the medial side of the distal end of the humerus.

Incision

Make a curved incision 8 cm to 10 cm long on the medial aspect of the elbow, centering the incision on the medial epicondyle (Fig. 3-7).

INTERNERVOUS PLANE

Proximally, the internervous plane lies between the brachialis (musculocutaneous nerve) and the triceps (radial nerve) (Fig. 3-8).

Distally, the plane lies between the brachialis (musculocutaneous nerve) and the pronator teres (median nerve) (see Fig. 3-8).

SUPERFICIAL SURGICAL DISSECTION

Palpate the ulnar nerve as it runs in its groove behind the medial condyle of the humerus. Incise the fascia over the nerve starting proximal to the medial epicondyle; then isolate the nerve along the length of the incision (Fig. 3-9).

Retract the anterior skin flap, together with the fascia overlying the pronator teres. The superficial flexor muscles of the forearm are now visible as they pass directly from their common origin on the medial epicondyle of the humerus (Fig. 3-10).

Define the interval between the pronator teres and the brachialis, taking care not to damage the median nerve, which enters the pronator teres near the midline. Gently retract the pronator teres medially, lifting it off the brachialis (Fig. 3-11). Make sure that the ulnar nerve is retracted inferiorly; then osteotomize the medial epicondyle. Reflect the epicondyle with its attached flexors distally, avoiding traction that might damage the median or anterior interosseous nerves. Superiorly, continue the dissection between the brachialis, retracting it anteriorly, and the triceps, retracting it posteriorly (Fig. 3-12).

FIG. 3-6. Position on the operating table.

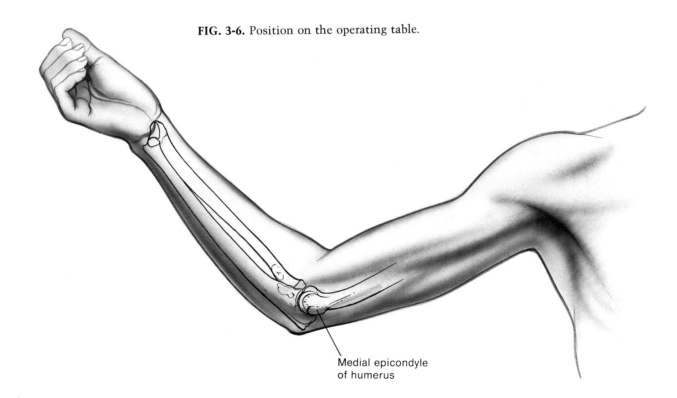

Medial epicondyle
of humerus

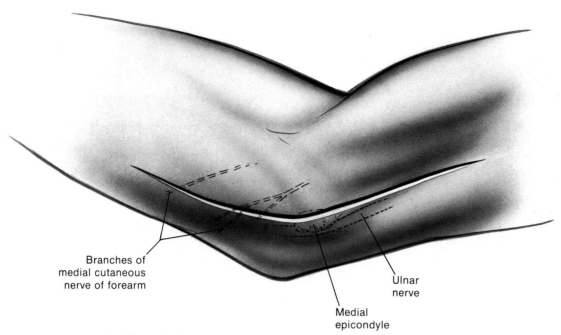

FIG. 3-7. Incision for the medial approach to the elbow, centered on the medial epicondyle.

FIG. 3-8. Internervous plane. Proximally, the plane is between the brachialis (musculocutaneous nerve) and the triceps (radial nerve); distally, it is between the brachialis and the pronator teres (median nerve).

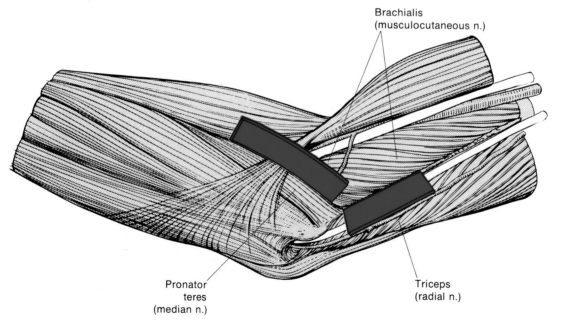

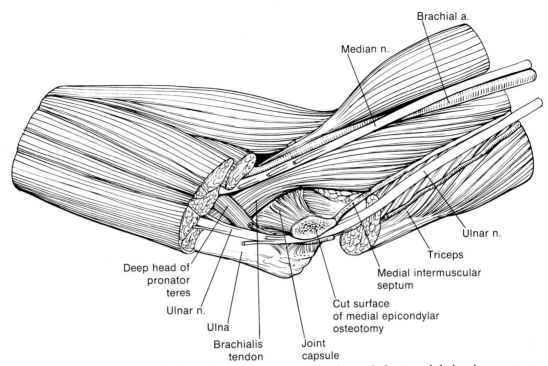

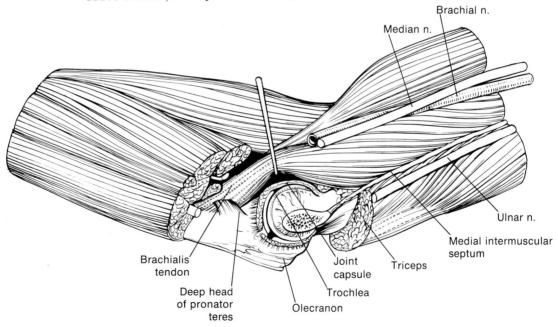

FIG. 3-36. The flexor muscles have been further resected. The medial epicondyle has been osteoto-mized. Distally, the ulnar nerve crosses the forearm between the flexor carpi ulnaris and the pro-fundus. The median nerve enters the forearm between the two heads of the pronator teres, lying on the tendon of the brachialis.

FIG. 3-37. The joint capsule has been opened. The brachialis is elevated from the capsule.

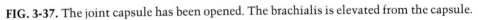

(For a discussion of the *brachialis*, see p. 67.)
For a discussion of the *biceps brachii*, see pp. 18-21.)

In front of the elbow, the biceps brachii develops a flat tendon, which also overlies the brachialis. The tendon rotates so that its anterior surface faces laterally as it passes between the two bones of the forearm before inserting into the back of the radius at the bicipital tuberosity. A bursa separates the tendon from the anterior part of the tuberosity.

As the biceps tendon crosses the front of the elbow, it gives off fibrous tissue from its medial side. This *bicipital aponeurosis*, or *lacertus fibrosus*, sweeps across the forearm by way of the deep fascia to insert into the subcutaneous border of the upper end of the ulna.

The bicipital aponeurosis forms part of the roof of the cubital fossa. It separates superficial nerves and vessels from deep ones. Lying superficial are the median cephalic vein, the median basilic vein, and the medial cutaneous nerve of the forearm.

Lying deep are the median nerve and the brachial artery.

The relationship of the median nerve, brachial artery, and brachial vein are easily remembered through the mnemonic VAN—Vein, Artery, Nerve—that labels the structures from the lateral to the medial aspect. All of them pass medial to the biceps tendon under the lacertus fibrosus (see Figs. 4-17 through 4-23).

APPLIED SURGICAL ANATOMY OF THE POSTERIOR APPROACH

(See Figs. 3-38 through 3-41.)

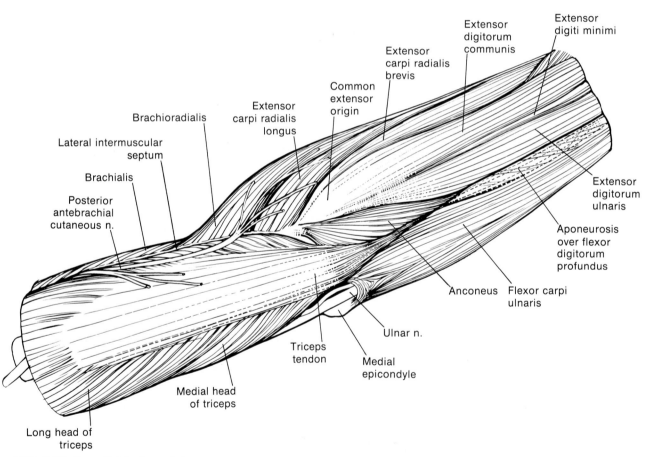

FIG. 3-38. Superficial view of the posterior aspect of the elbow. The triangular aponeurosis of the triceps runs down to its triangular insertion into the ulna. The ulnar nerve lies in its groove on the posterior aspect of the elbow. The brachial cutaneous nerve crosses the intermuscular septum on the posterior aspect of the elbow.

Anconeus. *Origin.* Lateral epicondyle of humerus and posterior joint capsule of elbow. *Insertion.* Lateral side of olecranon and posterior surface of ulna. *Action.* Extensor of elbow. *Nerve supply.* Radial nerve.

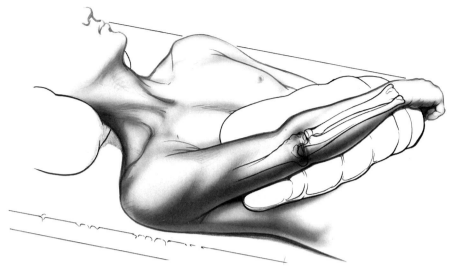

FIG. 4-18 Position of patient on the operating table, for exposure of the shaft of the ulna.

FIG. 4-19. Incision for ulnar exposure. Make a longitudinal incision over the subcutaneous border of the ulna.

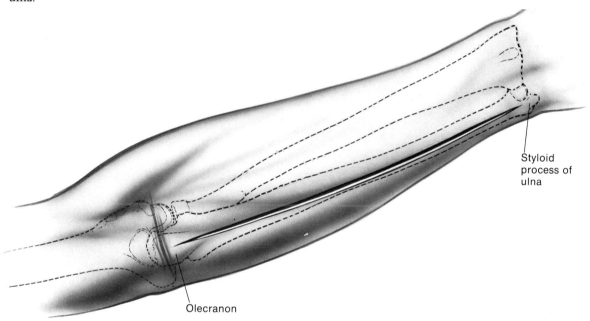

Styloid process of ulna

Olecranon

subperiosteally. If the dissection strays into the substance of the muscle, however, the nerve may be damaged. Because the nerve is most vulnerable during very proximal dissections, it should be identified as it passes through the two heads of flexor carpi ulnaris *before* the muscle is stripped off the proximal fifth of the bone (Fig. 4-23).

Vessels

The **ulnar artery** travels down the forearm with the ulnar nerve, lying on its radial side. Therefore, it is also vulnerable when dissection of the flexor carpi ulnaris is not carried out subperiosteally.

HOW TO ENLARGE THE APPROACH

Local Measures

The approach described gives excellent exposure of the entire bone and cannot be usefully enlarged by local measures.

Extensile Measures

The approach cannot be usefully extended distally. However, it can be extended over the olecranon and up the back of the arm, either to expose the elbow joint through an olecranon osteotomy or to approach the posterior aspect of the distal two thirds of the humerus.

125

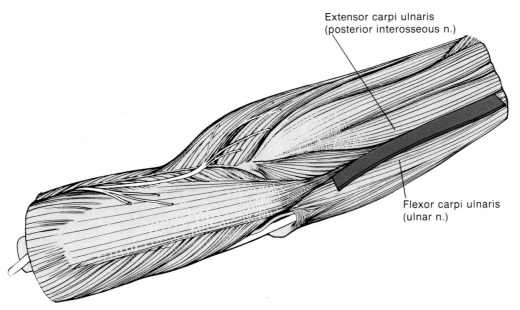

FIG. 4-20. The internervous plane lies between the extensor carpi ulnaris (posterior interosseous nerve) and the flexor carpi ulnaris (ulnar nerve).

FIG. 4-21. Make an incision through the fascia onto the subcutaneous border of the ulna.

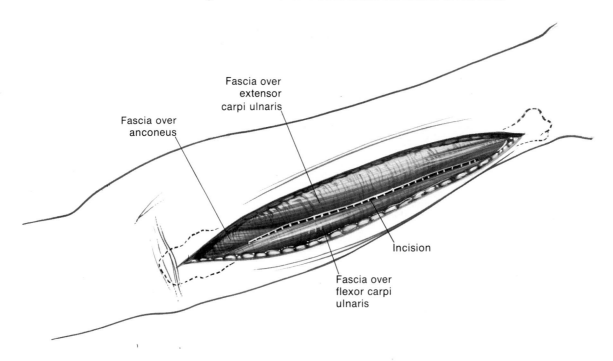

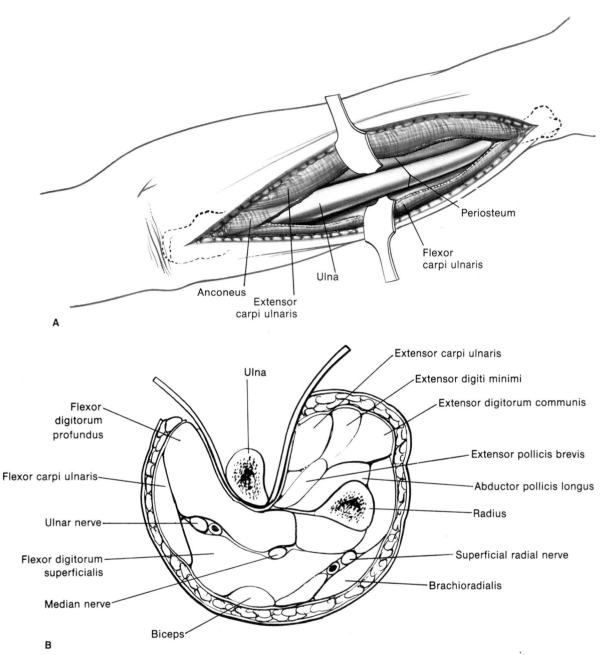

Periosteum

Flexor
carpi ulnaris

Ulna

Anconeus

Extensor
carpi ulnaris

A

Ulna

Extensor carpi ulnaris

Extensor digiti minimi

Extensor digitorum communis

Flexor
digitorum
profundus

Extensor pollicis brevis

Abductor pollicis longus

Flexor carpi ulnaris

Radius

Ulnar nerve

Flexor digitorum
superficialis

Superficial radial nerve

Median nerve

Brachioradialis

Biceps

B

FIG. 4-22. (**A**) Lift the periosteum longitudinally from the posterior aspect of the ulna, both radially and medially, to expose the entire posterior length of the ulna. (**B**) Subperiosteal dissection around the ulna is safe; the muscle masses on either side protect the vital structures.

APPLIED SURGICAL ANATOMY OF THE APPROACH TO THE ULNA

ANATOMY OF THE SURGICAL DISSECTION AND ITS DANGERS

Two muscles are separated in this approach: the flexor carpi ulnaris (ulnar nerve) and the extensor carpi ulnaris (posterior interosseous nerve) (see Fig. 4-23).

The muscular branch of the ulnar nerve, which innervates the flexor carpi ulnaris, effectively tethers the nerve, preventing further distal mobilization during decompression at the elbow. Compression lesions of the nerve have been described (see Fig. 3-40).[17,18]

The *extensor carpi ulnaris* is the most medial of the muscles innervated by the posterior interosseous nerve. It thus forms one border of the internervous plane between muscles innervated by the posterior interosseous nerve and those innervated by the ulnar nerve, the most medial of which is the flexor carpi ulnaris (see Fig. 4-20).

The *ulnar nerve* runs down the medial side of the forearm between the flexor digitorum profundus and the flexor digitorum superficialis and under the flexor carpi ulnaris. In the forearm, it supplies the flexor carpi ulnaris and the ulnar half of the flexor digitorum profundus (see Figs. 4-15 and 3-40).

The *ulnar artery* is a terminal branch of the brachial artery. It usually enters the forearm deep to the deep head of the pronator teres before angling medially across the forearm, passing under the fibrous arch of the flexor digitorum superficialis, where it runs just deep to the median nerve (see Figs. 4-13, 4-14, and 4-15). In the distal two thirds of the forearm, the artery runs on the lateral side of the ulnar nerve, lying on the flexor digitorum profundus and under the flexor carpi ulnaris. The artery has one major branch in the forearm, the common interosseous artery, which divides almost immediately into two tributaries, the anterior interosseous artery (which runs down the forearm in the midline, lying on the interosseous membrane) and the posterior interosseous artery (which pierces the interosseous membrane, running down the forearm in its posterior compartment) (see Fig. 4-15).

The ulnar nerve and ulnar artery may be endangered during superficial dissection if the dissection strays to the flexor side of the bone.

FIG. 4-23. The ulnar nerve is vulnerable during the most proximal dissections of the ulna. It must be identified before muscle is stripped from bone in the proximal fifth.

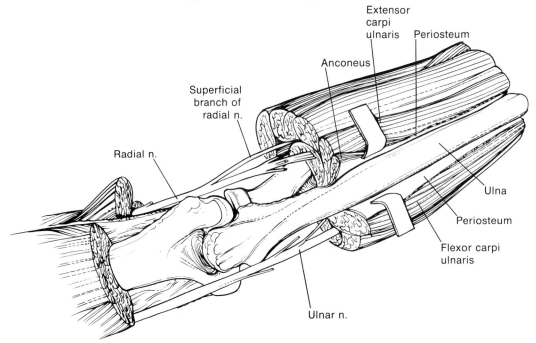

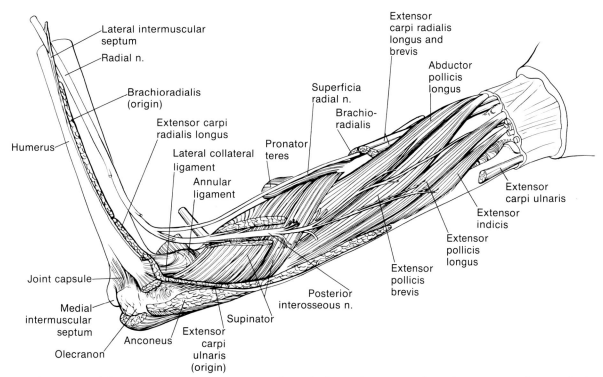

FIG. 4-34. The course of the posterior interosseous nerve through the supinator muscle, as it runs to supply muscles in the forearm.

Extensor Carpi Ulnaris. *Origin.* Common extensor origin on lateral epicondyle of humerus and subcutaneous border of ulna. (Shared origin with flexor carpi ulnaris.) *Insertion.* Base of fifth metacarpal. *Action.* Extensor and ulnar deviator of wrist. *Nerve supply.* Posterior interosseous nerve.

Extensor Digitorum Communis. *Origin.* Common extensor origin on lateral epicondyle of humerus. *Insertion.* Into extensor apparatus of fingers. *Action.* Extensor of wrist and fingers. *Nerve supply.* Posterior interosseous nerve.

Vessels

The **posterior interosseous artery** accompanies the posterior interosseous nerve as it runs along the interosseous membrane in the proximal two thirds of the forearm. The posterior interosseous artery enters the extensor compartment of the forearm by passing between the radius and the ulna through the interosseous membrane (Fig. 4-35). The artery then joins the posterior interosseous nerve distal to the distal edge of the deep head of the supinator muscle.

The posterior interosseous artery is too small to be easily dissected down to the level of the wrist. Most of the blood supply for the posterior area comes from an anterior interosseous artery via branches that perforate the interosseous membrane. The tendons running in this area may have a marginal blood supply.

Although the artery may be damaged during the posterior approach to the radius, good collateral circulation appears to protect the extremity from any functional deficits.

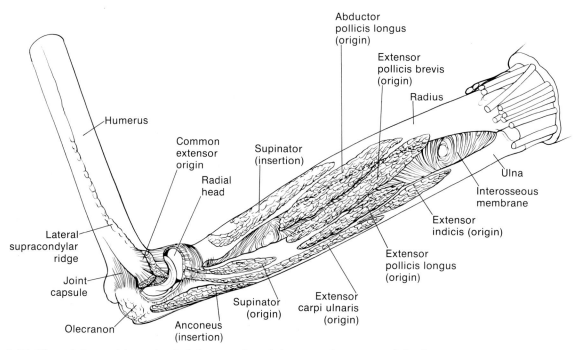

FIG. 4-35. The origins and insertions of the muscles of the posterior aspect of the forearm.

Extensor Carpi Radialis Longus. *Origin.* Lower third of lateral supracondylar ridge of humerus, lateral intermuscular septum of arm. *Insertion.* Base of second metacarpal. *Action.* Extensor and radial deviator of wrist. *Nerve supply.* Radial nerve.

Extenor Carpi Radialis Brevis. *Origin.* Common extensor origin on lateral epicondyle of humerus and radial collateral ligament of elbow. *Insertion.* Base of third metacarpal. *Action.* Extensor and radial deviator of wrist. *Nerve supply.* Radial nerve (superficial radial nerve).

Supinator. *Origin.* From two heads. Superficial head: from lateral epicondyle of humerus, lateral collateral ligament of elbow, and supinator crest of ulna. Deep head: from supinator crest and fossa of ulna. *Insertion.* Anterior aspect of radius. *Action.* Supinator of forearm. Weak flexor of elbow. *Nerve supply.* Posterior interosseous nerve.

Extensor Pollicis Longus. *Origin.* Posterior surface of ulna in its middle third and from interosseous membrane. *Insertion.* Distal phalanx of thumb. *Action.* Extensor of thumb and wrist. *Nerve supply.* Posterior interosseous nerve.

Abductor Pollicis Longus. *Origin.* Posterior surface of ulna, posterior interosseous membrane, and middle third of posterior surface of radius. *Insertion.* Base of thumb, metacarpal. *Action.* Abductor and extensor of thumb. *Nerve supply.* Posterior interosseous nerve.

Extensor Pollicis Brevis. *Origin.* Posterior surface of radius and interosseous membrane. *Insertion.* Base of proximal phalanx of thumb. *Action.* Extensor of proximal phalanx of thumb. *Nerve supply.* Posterior interosseous nerve.

Extensor Indicis. *Origin.* Posterior surface of ulnar shaft and interosseous membrane. *Insertion.* Extensor apparatus of index finger via ulnar side of tendon of extensor digitorum that runs to index finger. *Action.* Extensor of index finger. *Nerve supply.* Posterior interosseous nerve.

Extensor Digiti Minimi. *Origin.* Common extensor origin on lateral epicondyle of humerus. *Insertion.* Extensor apparatus of little finger. *Action.* Extensor of little finger. *Nerve supply.* Posterior interosseous nerve.

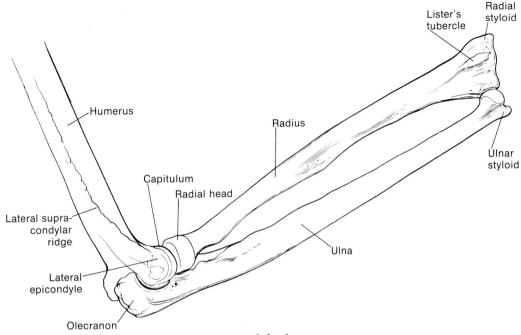

FIG. 4-36. The bones of the posterior aspect of the forearm.

REFERENCES

1. HENRY AK: Extensile Exposure, 2nd ed, pp. 100–106. Baltimore, Williams & Wilkins, 1970
2. STRAUB LB: Congenital absence of the ulna. Am J Surg 109:300, 1965
3. SPINNER M: Injuries to the Major Branches of Peripheral Nerves of the Forearm, 2nd ed. Philadelphia, WB Saunders, 1978
4. MULLER ME, ALLGONER M, WILLENGER H: Manual of Internal Fixation. New York, Springer-Verlag, 1970
5. FROHSE F, FRANKEL M: Die Muskeln Des Menschlichen Armes. In Bardelehen's Handbuch der Anatomie des Menschlichen. Jena, Fisher, 1980
6. CAPENER N: Posterior interosseous nerve lesions: Proceedings of the second hand club. J Bone Joint Surg (Br) 46:361, 1964
7. SHARRARD WJW: Posterior interosseous neuritis. J Bone Joint Surg (Br) 48:777, 1966
8. WEINBERGER LM: Non-traumatic paralysis of the dorsal interosseous nerve. Surg Gynecol Obstet 69:358, 1939
9. ROLES NC, MAUDSLET RH: Radial tunnel syndrome: Resistant tennis elbow as a nerve entrapment. J Bone Joint Surg (Br) 54:499, 1972
10. SOLNITZKY O: Pronator syndrome: Compression neuropathy of the median nerve at level of pronator teres muscle. Georgetown Med Bull 13:232, 1960
11. KOPELL HP, THOMPSON WAL: Pronator syndrome. N Engl J Med 239: 713, 1958
12. SPINNER M: Injuries to the Major Branches of Peripheral Nerves of the Forearm, 2nd ed, pp. 195–196. Philadelphia, WB Saunders, 1978
13. KILOH LG, NEKN S: Isolated neuritis of the anterior interosseous nerve. Br Med J 1:850, 1952
14. SPINNER M: The anterior interosseous nerve syndrome, with special attention to its variations. J Bone Joint Surg (Am) 54A:84, 1970
15. FEARN CB, GOODFELLOW JW: Anterior interosseous nerve palsy. J Bone Joint Surg (Br) 47:91 (February) 1965
16. ARMISTEAD RB, LINSCHEID RL, DOBYNS JH et al: Ulnar lengthening in the treatment of Kienböck's disease. J Bone Joint Surg (Am) 64:170, 1982
17. OSBORNE G: Compression neuritis at the elbow. Hand Z:10, 1970
18. VANDERPOOL DW, CHALMERS J, LAMB DW et al: Peripheral compression lesions of the ulnar nerve. J Bone Joint Surg (Br) 50:792, 1968
19. THOMPSON JE: Anatomical methods of approach in operations on the long bones of the extremities. Ann Surg 68:309, 1918
20. SPINNER M: The arcade of Frohse and its relationship to posterior interosseous nerve paralysis. J Bone Joint Surg (Br) 50:809, 1968
21. DAVIES F, LAIRD M: The supinator muscle and the deep radial (posterior interosseous) nerve. Anat Rec 101:243, 1948
22. SALSBURY CR: The nerve to extensor carpi radialis brevis. Br J Surg 26:9597, 1938
23. SPINNER O: Management of peripheral nerve problems. In Management of Nerve Compression Lesions of the Upper Extremity, p 569, Chap 34. Philadelphia, WB Saunders, 1980

5

The Wrist and Hand

Seven approaches to the wrist and hand are described: three each to the wrist, flexor tendons, and scaphoid.

The *dorsal approach to the wrist joint* is used mainly in rheumatoid arthritis and for work on the bones of the carpus; the *volar approach* is used mainly for exploration of the carpal tunnel and its enclosed structures. The applied anatomy of each approach is considered separately.

The *volar approach to the flexor tendons* is the most common. It also gives excellent exposure of the digital nerves and vessels. The *midlateral approach* is useful in the treatment of phalangeal fractures. The applied anatomy of the finger flexor tendons follows these two approaches.

Dorsal and volar approaches to the scaphoid are described together, with a brief description of the blood supply of that bone.

Infection within the hand is a common clinical problem. The methods of drainage for these conditions are described together, with an introducton on the general principles of drainage in the hand. Of all the infections requiring surgery, paronychia and felons are by far the most common.

Throughout this book, we have related anatomy to surgical approaches. In the hand, however, the majority of wounds encountered arise from trauma, not from planned incisions. A brief review of the overall anatomy of the hand is vital to explain the damage that may be caused by a particular injury. Although clinical findings are the key to accurate diagnosis of tissue trauma, knowledge of the underlying anatomy is crucial to bringing to light all possibilities and minimizes the risk of overlooking a significant injury. For example, arterial hemorrhage from a digital artery in a finger is nearly always associated with damage to a digital nerve, since the nerve lies volar to the severed artery. Arterial hemorrhage in a finger should alert the surgeon to the possibility of nerve injury, which often appears clinically as a change in the quality of sensation rather than as complete anesthesia and can be missed in a brief examination.

Therefore, the chapter ends with a section on the topographical anatomy of the hand. The anatomy is considered in one section—and not on an approach-by-approach basis—to give a clear and integrated picture of hand anatomy.

DORSAL APPROACH TO THE WRIST

The dorsal approach gives excellent exposure of all the extensor tendons that pass over the dorsal surface of the wrist. It also allows access to the dorsal aspect of the wrist itself, the dorsal aspect of the carpus, and the dorsal surface of the proximal ends of the middle metacarpals. Its uses include the following:

1. Synovectomy and repair of the extensor tendons in cases of rheumatoid arthritis; dorsal stabilization of the wrist[1,2]
2. Wrist fusion[3]
3. Excision of the lower end of the radius for benign or malignant tumors
4. Open reduction and internal fixation of certain distal radial and carpal fractures and dislocations, including dorsal metacarpal dislocations, displaced intra-articular dorsal lip fractures of the radius, and transscaphoid perilunate dislocations
5. Proximal row carpectomy[4,5]

POSITION OF PATIENT

Place the patient supine on the operating table. Pronate the forearm and put the arm on an arm

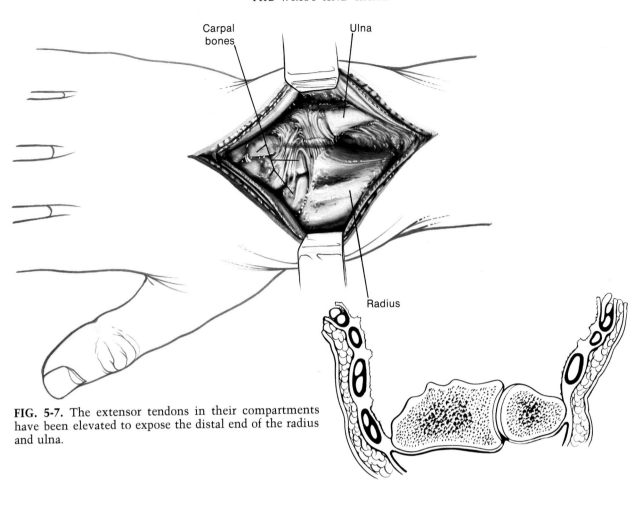

FIG. 5-7. The extensor tendons in their compartments have been elevated to expose the distal end of the radius and ulna.

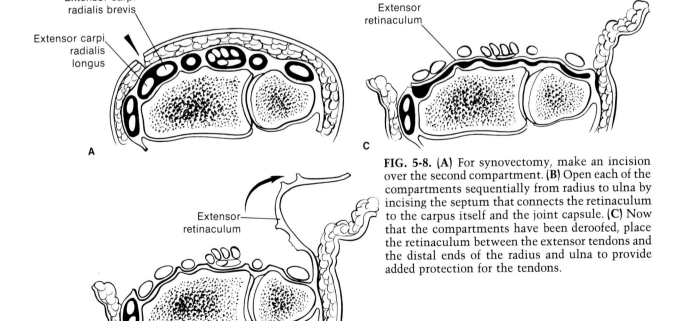

FIG. 5-8. (A) For synovectomy, make an incision over the second compartment. (B) Open each of the compartments sequentially from radius to ulna by incising the septum that connects the retinaculum to the carpus itself and the joint capsule. (C) Now that the compartments have been deroofed, place the retinaculum between the extensor tendons and the distal ends of the radius and ulna to provide added protection for the tendons.

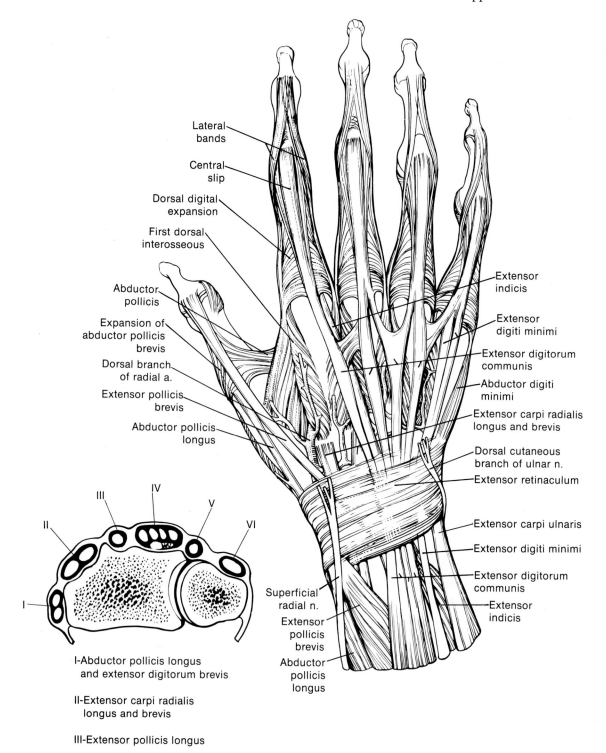

Lateral bands

Central slip

Dorsal digital expansion

First dorsal interosseous

Abductor pollicis

Expansion of abductor pollicis brevis

Dorsal branch of radial a.

Extensor pollicis brevis

Abductor pollicis longus

Extensor indicis

Extensor digiti minimi

Extensor digitorum communis

Abductor digiti minimi

Extensor carpi radialis longus and brevis

Dorsal cutaneous branch of ulnar n.

Extensor retinaculum

Extensor carpi ulnaris

Extensor digiti minimi

Extensor digitorum communis

Extensor indicis

Superficial radial n.

Extensor pollicis brevis

Abductor pollicis longus

I-Abductor pollicis longus and extensor digitorum brevis

II-Extensor carpi radialis longus and brevis

III-Extensor pollicis longus

IV-Extensor digitorum communis and extensor indicis

V-Extensor digiti minimi

VI-Extensor carpi ulnaris

FIG. 5-9. The dorsal aspect of the wrist and hand. *(Inset)* Cross section of the distal forearm. Note the compartmentalization of tendons into six distinct tunnels at the dorsal aspect of the distal forearm.

DANGERS

Nerves

The **radial nerve** (superficial radial nerve) emerges from beneath the tendon of the brachioradialis just above the wrist joint before traveling to the dorsum of the hand. The skin incision lies between skin supplied by cutaneous branches of the ulnar nerve and skin supplied by cutaneous branches of the radial nerve. Damage to cutaneous nerves occurs only if you begin dissecting within the fat. If you take the incision down to the extensor retinaculum before elevating the ulnar and radial flaps, the nerves are protected by the full thickness of the fat (see Fig. 5-9).

Cutting a cutaneous nerve may result in a painful neuroma; the resultant sensory defect is rarely significant.

Vessels

The **radial artery** crosses the wrist joint on its lateral aspect. As long as the dissection at the level of the wrist joint remains subperiosteal, the artery is difficult to damage.

HOW TO ENLARGE THE APPROACH

Because it does not make use of an internervous plane, the incision cannot be extended proximally to expose the rest of the radius. However, you can extend it to expose the distal half of the dorsal aspect of the radius by retracting the abductor pollicis longus and the extensor pollicis brevis, which cross the operative field obliquely.

To expose the entire dorsal surface of the metacarpals, extend the incision distally and retract the extensor tendons. (This type of extension is seldom required in practice.) The approach gives excellent exposure of the wrist joint and allows easy access to all six compartments of the extensor tunnel.

APPLIED SURGICAL ANATOMY OF THE DORSAL APPROACH TO THE WRIST

OVERVIEW

Twelve tendons cross the dorsal aspect of the wrist joint and pass beneath the extensor retinaculum, a thickening of the deep fascia of the forearm. The extensor retinaculum prevents the tendons from bowstringing. Fibrous septa pass from the deep surface of the retinaculum to the bones of the forearm, dividing the extensor tunnel into six compartments. These septa must be separated from the retinaculum so that each compartment can be opened in surgery (Fig. 5-9).

LANDMARKS AND INCISION

Landmarks

Two bony landmarks lie on the dorsal aspect of the wrist. The *styloid process* is the distal end of the lateral side of the radius. It is also the site of attachment of the tendon of the brachioradialis. Its medial part articulates with the scaphoid bone (see Fig. 5-12A). Strong and sudden radial deviation of the wrist may cause the radial styloid process to slam into the scaphoid and fracture it (see Fig. 5-12B).

The styloid process is often excised when the scaphoid fails to reunite or after arthritic changes in the wrist joint have affected the radial margin of the radioscaphoid joint.

Lister's tubercle (dorsoradial tubercle) is a small bony prominence on the dorsum of the radius. The tendon of the extensor pollicis longus angles around its distal end, changing direction about 45° as it does so. When the wrist is hyperextended, the base of the third metacarpal comes very close to Lister's tubercle and the two bones can crush the trapped tendon of the extensor pollicis longus. That is probably why the tendon suffers delayed rupture in some cases of minimal or undisplaced fractures of the distal radius; the tendon sustains a vascular insult at the time of the original injury, even though it remains intact (see Fig. 5-12C).[4]

Incision

Longitudinal incisions crossing the lines of cleavage of the skin almost perpendicularly on the dorsum of the wrist can cause broad scarring. Nevertheless, because the skin on the wrist is so loose, this is one of those rare occasions when a skin incision *can* cross a major skin crease at right angles without causing a joint contracture.

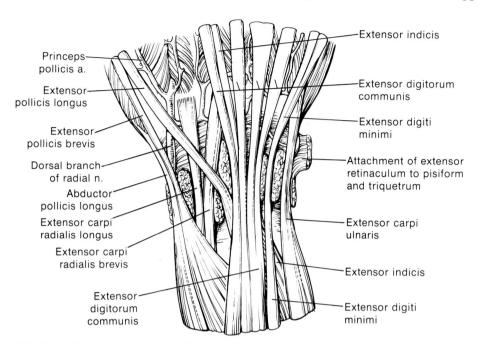

FIG. 5-10. Anatomy of the distal forearm, with the extensor retinaculum excised and the septa remaining. The retinaculum on the ulnar side inserts into the triquetrum and pisiform bones.

SUPERFICIAL AND DEEP SURGICAL DISSECTION

The extensor retinaculum is a narrow (2-cm) fibrous band that lies obliquely across the dorsal aspect of the wrist. Its radial side is attached to the anterolateral border of the radius; its ulnar border is attached to the pisiform and triquetral bones. (Were it attached to both bones of the forearm instead, pronation and supination would be impossible, because its fibrous tissue is incapable of stretching the necessary 30%.)

Fibrous septa pass from the deep surface of the extensor retinaculum to the bones of the carpus, dividing the extensor tunnel into six compartments (Fig. 5-10). From the radial (lateral) to the ulnar (medial) aspect, the compartments contain the following:

1. *Abductor pollicis longus and extensor pollicis brevis.* These tendons lie over the lateral aspect of the radius. They may become trapped or inflamed beneath the extensor retinaculum in their fibro-osseous canal, producing De Quervain's syndrome (stenosing tenosynovitis).

2. *Extensor carpi radialis longus and extensor carpi radialis brevis.* These muscles run on the radial side of Lister's tubercle before reaching the dorsum of the hand. The tendon of the extensor carpi radialis longus is frequently used in tendon transfers.

3. *Extensor pollicis longus.* This tendon passes into the dorsum of the hand on the ulnar side of Lister's tubercle. It may rupture in association with fractures or rheumatoid arthritis.

4. *Extensor digitorum communis and extensor indicis.* The indicis tendon is frequently used in tendon transfers.

5. *Extensor digiti minimi.* This tendon overlies the distal radioulnar joint.

6. *Extensor carpi ulnaris.* This tendon passes near the base of the ulnar styloid process. It is sometimes used in tendon transfers (Fig. 5-11; see Fig. 5-10).

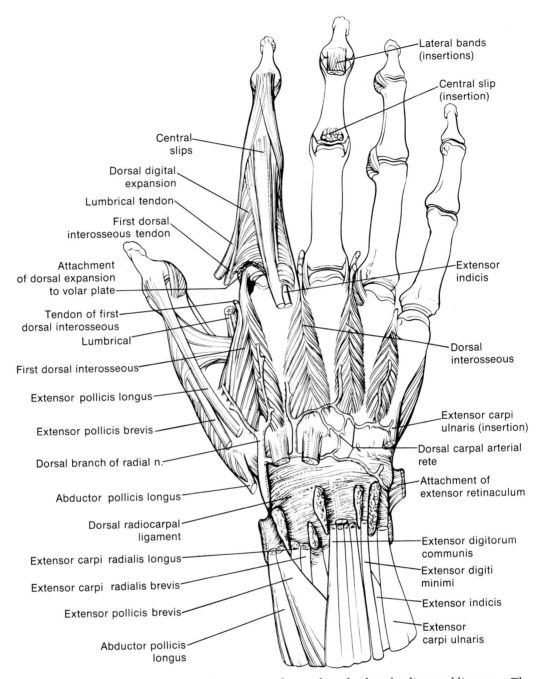

FIG 5-11. The extensor tendons have been removed, revealing the dorsal radiocarpal ligament. The radial artery is seen piercing the first dorsal interosseus muscle and contributing to the dorsal carpal rete. Note the hood mechanism for the index finger; contributions are made to it by the first dorsal interosseus and the first lumbrical.

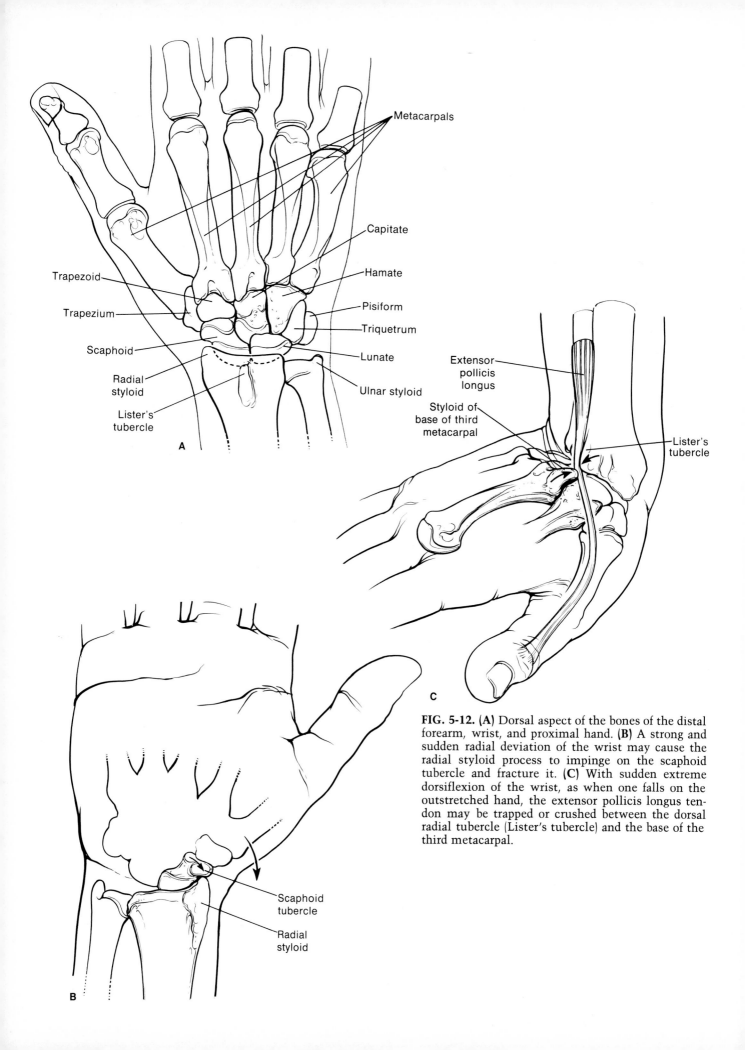

FIG. 5-12. (A) Dorsal aspect of the bones of the distal forearm, wrist, and proximal hand. **(B)** A strong and sudden radial deviation of the wrist may cause the radial styloid process to impinge on the scaphoid tubercle and fracture it. **(C)** With sudden extreme dorsiflexion of the wrist, as when one falls on the outstretched hand, the extensor pollicis longus tendon may be trapped or crushed between the dorsal radial tubercle (Lister's tubercle) and the base of the third metacarpal.

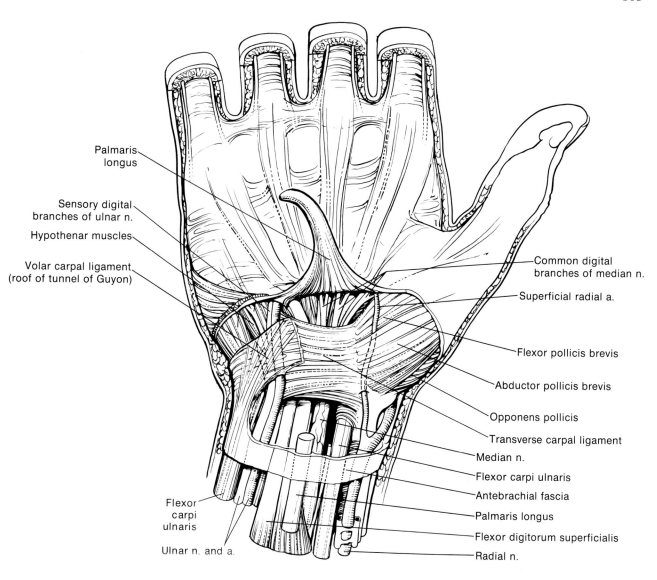

Palmaris longus

Sensory digital branches of ulnar n.

Hypothenar muscles

Volar carpal ligament (roof of tunnel of Guyon)

Common digital branches of median n.

Superficial radial a.

Flexor pollicis brevis

Abductor pollicis brevis

Opponens pollicis

Transverse carpal ligament

Median n.

Flexor carpi ulnaris

Antebrachial fascia

Palmaris longus

Flexor digitorum superficialis

Radial n.

Flexor carpi ulnaris

Ulnar n. and a.

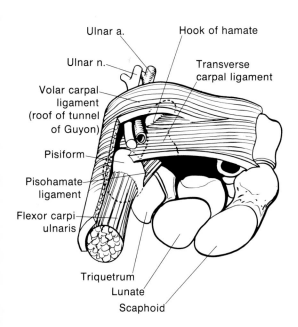

Ulnar a.

Hook of hamate

Ulnar n.

Transverse carpal ligament

Volar carpal ligament (roof of tunnel of Guyon)

Pisiform

Pisohamate ligament

Flexor carpi ulnaris

Triquetrum

Lunate

Scaphoid

FIG. 5-31. The palmar aponeurosis and fascia have been elevated to reveal the transverse carpal ligament. The fascia of the forearm and the expansions of the flexor carpi ulnaris (volar carpal ligament) are left intact where they form the roof of the tunnel of Guyon. *(Inset)* The canal of Guyon looking from proximal to distal. The transverse carpal ligament forms the floor of the tunnel of Guyon; the roof is formed by the volar carpal ligament, which is a condensation of the fascia of the forearm and expansions of the flexor carpi ulnaris tendon. Medially, the canal is formed by the pisiform and laterally by the hook of the hamate bone.

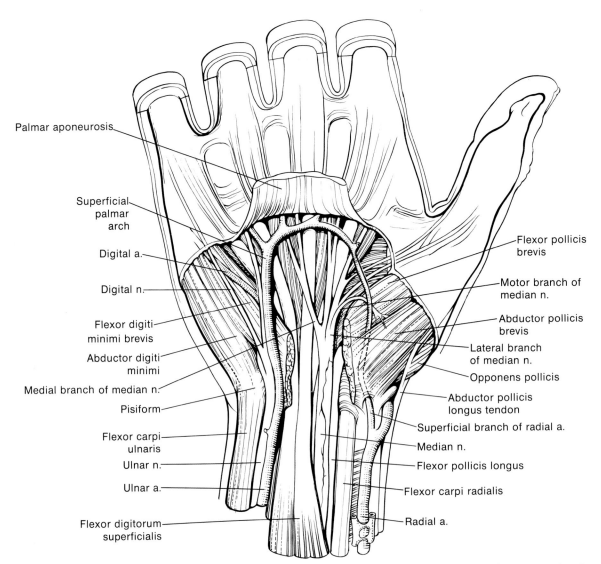

Palmar aponeurosis

Superficial palmar arch

Digital a.

Digital n.

Flexor digiti minimi brevis

Abductor digiti minimi

Medial branch of median n.

Pisiform

Flexor carpi ulnaris

Ulnar n.

Ulnar a.

Flexor digitorum superficialis

Flexor pollicis brevis

Motor branch of median n.

Abductor pollicis brevis

Lateral branch of median n.

Opponens pollicis

Abductor pollicis longus tendon

Superficial branch of radial a.

Median n.

Flexor pollicis longus

Flexor carpi radialis

Radial a.

FIG. 5-32. The palmar aponeurosis has been resected farther distally to expose the superficial palmar arterial arch. The transverse carpal ligament has also been resected. The median nerve lies superficial to the tendons of the profundus but at the same level with the superficialis muscle tendons. Note the motor branch of the median nerve to the thenar muscles. The location of its division from the median nerve is quite variable.

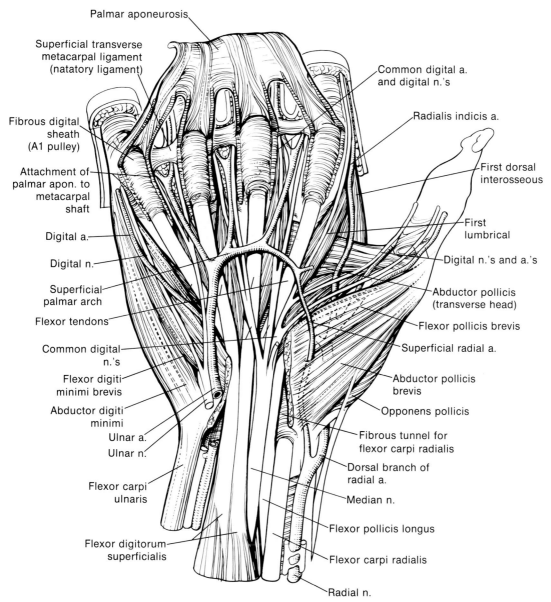

Palmar aponeurosis

Superficial transverse
metacarpal ligament
(natatory ligament)

Fibrous digital
sheath
(A1 pulley)

Attachment of
palmar apon. to
metacarpal
shaft

Digital a.

Digital n.

Superficial
palmar arch

Flexor tendons

Common digital
n.'s

Flexor digiti
minimi brevis

Abductor digiti
minimi

Ulnar a.

Ulnar n.

Flexor carpi
ulnaris

Flexor digitorum
superficialis

Common digital a.
and digital n.'s

Radialis indicis a.

First dorsal
interosseous

First
lumbrical

Digital n.'s and a.'s

Abductor pollicis
(transverse head)

Flexor pollicis brevis

Superficial radial a.

Abductor pollicis
brevis

Opponens pollicis

Fibrous tunnel for
flexor carpi radialis

Dorsal branch of
radial a.

Median n.

Flexor pollicis longus

Flexor carpi radialis

Radial n.

FIG. 5-33. The palmar aponeurosis has been elevated up to its attachment to the digital flexor sheaths. Its deeper attachments to the carpal plate and bone have been cut. The flexor tendons and digital nerves are shown in continuity, as are the superficial palmar arch and the thenar and hyperthenar muscles. Note that the digital nerves and vessels go deep or dorsal to the natatory ligaments.

Flexor Pollicis Brevis. *Origin.* Flexor retinaculum. *Insertion.* Radial border of proximal phalanx of thumb. *Action.* Flexor of metacarpophalangeal joint of thumb. *Nerve supply.* Median nerve (motor or recurrent branch).

Abductor Pollicis Brevis. *Origin.* Flexor retinaculum and tubercle of scaphoid. *Insertion.* Radial side of base of proximal phalanx of thumb. *Action.* Abduction of thumb at metacarpophalangeal joint and rotation of proximal phalanx of thumb. *Nerve supply.* Median nerve (motor or recurrent branch).

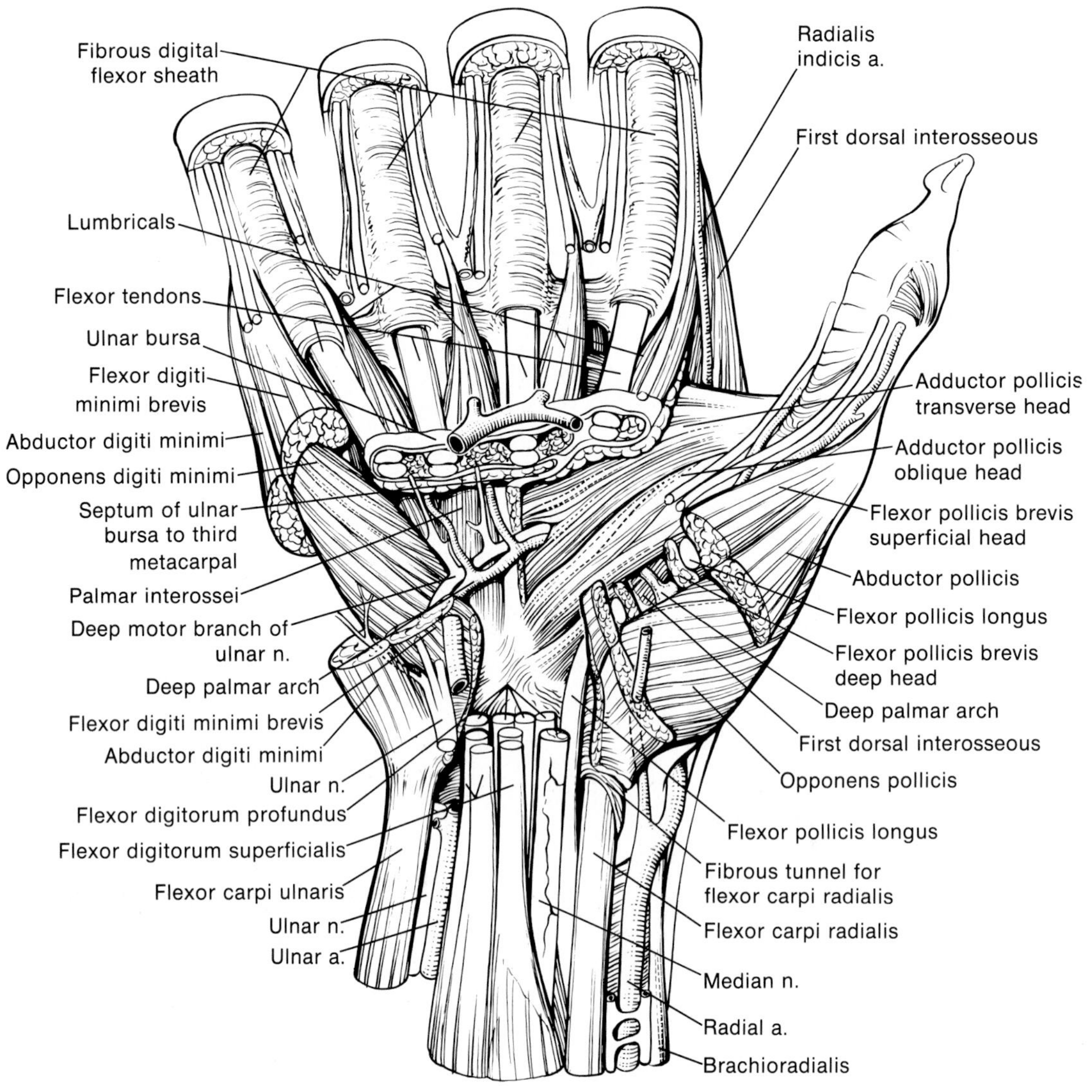
Fibrous digital flexor sheath
Radialis indicis a.
First dorsal interosseous
Lumbricals
Flexor tendons
Ulnar bursa
Flexor digiti minimi brevis
Abductor digiti minimi
Opponens digiti minimi
Septum of ulnar bursa to third metacarpal
Palmar interossei
Deep motor branch of ulnar n.
Deep palmar arch
Flexor digiti minimi brevis
Abductor digiti minimi
Ulnar n.
Flexor digitorum profundus
Flexor digitorum superficialis
Flexor carpi ulnaris
Ulnar n.
Ulnar a.
Adductor pollicis transverse head
Adductor pollicis oblique head
Flexor pollicis brevis superficial head
Abductor pollicis
Flexor pollicis longus
Flexor pollicis brevis deep head
Deep palmar arch
First dorsal interosseous
Opponens pollicis
Flexor pollicis longus
Fibrous tunnel for flexor carpi radialis
Flexor carpi radialis
Median n.
Radial a.
Brachioradialis

FIG. 5-34. Portions of the thenar and hyperthenar muscles have been resected to reveal their layering. The ulnar nerve passes between the origin of the abductor digiti minimi and the flexor digiti minimi. In the thenar region, the course of the flexor pollicis longus is seen as it crosses between the two heads of the flexor pollicis brevis. Portions of the long flexors of the fingers have been resected to show their layering: The superficial palmar arch runs superficial to the tendons, while the deep palmar arch is immediately deep to the tendons. Note that potential spaces develop on the undersurface of the flexor tendons and their sheaths and the deep intrinsic muscles of the hand, the interosseus on the hyperthenar side and the adductor pollicis on the thenar side. A septum that runs from the undersurface of the flexor tendons to the third metacarpal divides the two spaces. More distally, the superficial transverse ligament has been resected, revealing the course of the lumbricals and the digital vessels that run superficial or palmar to the deep transverse metacarpal ligaments.

Adductor Pollicis. *Origin.* Oblique head from bases of second and third metacarpals, trapezoid, and capitate. Transverse head from palmar border of third metacarpal. *Insertion.* Ulnar side of base of proximal phalanx of thumb via ulnar sesamoid. *Action.* Adduction of thumb. Opposition of thumb. *Nerve supply.* Deep branch of ulnar nerve.

Opponens Pollicis. *Origin.* Flexor retinaculum. *Insertion.* Radial border of thumb metacarpal. *Action.* Opposition of metacarpal bone of thumb. *Nerve supply.* Median nerve (motor or recurrent branch).

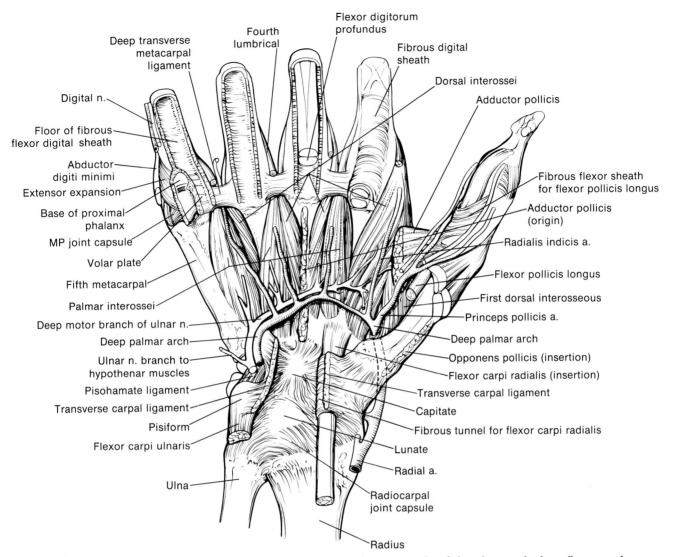

Deep transverse metacarpal ligament — **Fourth lumbrical** — **Flexor digitorum profundus** — **Fibrous digital sheath** — **Dorsal interossei** — **Adductor pollicis**

Digital n.

Floor of fibrous flexor digital sheath

Abductor digiti minimi

Extensor expansion

Base of proximal phalanx

MP joint capsule

Volar plate

Fifth metacarpal

Palmar interossei

Deep motor branch of ulnar n.

Deep palmar arch

Ulnar n. branch to hypothenar muscles

Pisohamate ligament

Transverse carpal ligament

Pisiform

Flexor carpi ulnaris

Ulna

Fibrous flexor sheath for flexor pollicis longus

Adductor pollicis (origin)

Radialis indicis a.

Flexor pollicis longus

First dorsal interosseous

Princeps pollicis a.

Deep palmar arch

Opponens pollicis (insertion)

Flexor carpi radialis (insertion)

Transverse carpal ligament

Capitate

Fibrous tunnel for flexor carpi radialis

Lunate

Radial a.

Radiocarpal joint capsule

Radius

FIG. 5-35. The deepest layer of the palm is revealed. The deep palmar arterial arch lies deep to the long flexor tendon and superficial to the interosseus muscles. It crosses the palm with the deep branch (motor branch) of the ulnar nerve. The nerve supplies all of the interosseous muscles. More distal, the interosseous muscles are seen running deep (dorsal) to the deep transverse ligament. The deep transverse metacarpal ligaments attach to the palmar plate, which is seen on the fifth metacarpal. The pulleys of the thumb are seen in relationship to the digital nerves.

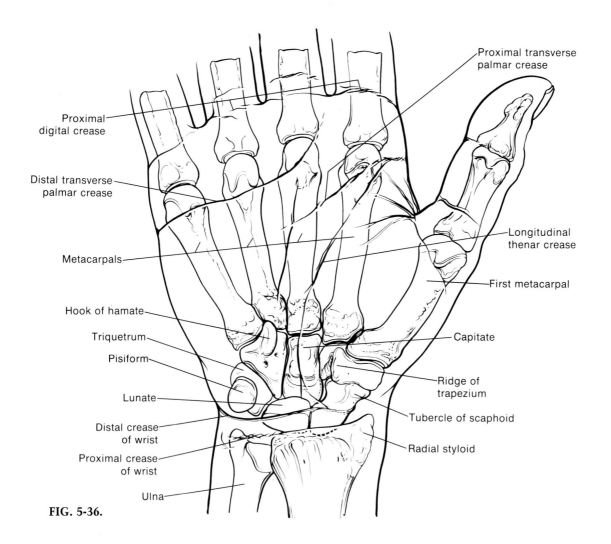

Proximal digital crease

Distal transverse palmar crease

Metacarpals

Hook of hamate

Triquetrum

Pisiform

Lunate

Distal crease of wrist

Proximal crease of wrist

Ulna

Proximal transverse palmar crease

Longitudinal thenar crease

First metacarpal

Capitate

Ridge of trapezium

Tubercle of scaphoid

Radial styloid

FIG. 5-36.

FIG. 5-36A.

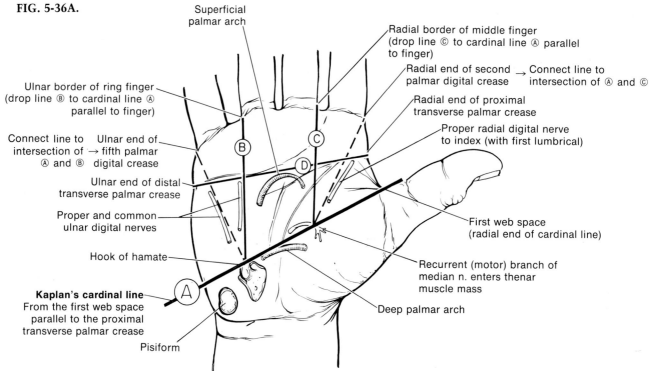

Superficial palmar arch

Ulnar border of ring finger (drop line ⑧ to cardinal line Ⓐ parallel to finger)

Connect line to   Ulnar end of
intersection of → fifth palmar
Ⓐ and ⑧   digital crease

Ulnar end of distal transverse palmar crease

Proper and common ulnar digital nerves

Hook of hamate

Kaplan's cardinal line
From the first web space parallel to the proximal transverse palmar crease

Pisiform

Radial border of middle finger (drop line Ⓒ to cardinal line Ⓐ parallel to finger)

Radial end of second → Connect line to
palmar digital crease   intersection of Ⓐ and Ⓒ

Radial end of proximal transverse palmar crease

Proper radial digital nerve to index (with first lumbrical)

First web space (radial end of cardinal line)

Recurrent (motor) branch of median n. enters thenar muscle mass

Deep palmar arch

1. Recurrent motor branch of median nerve Ⓐ Ⓒ
2. Superficial palmar arch Ⓓ
3. Deep palmar arch Ⓐ
4. Proper radial digital nerve to index—Radial dotted line

5. (a) Proper ulnar digital nerve—Ulnar dotted line
   (b) Common ulnar digital nerve ⑧
6. Hook of hamate Ⓐ + ⑧
7. Pisiform Ⓐ

FIG. 5-36. The bones of the wrist and palm and proximal metacarpals are seen in relationship to the creases of the wrist. The necks of the metacarpals are at the level of the distal palmar crease. The distal wrist crease runs from the proximal portion of the pisiform to the proximal portion of the tubercle of the scaphoid and marks the proximal level of the volar carpal ligament. The proximal transverse palmar crease is at the radiocarpal joint.

VOLAR APPROACH TO THE FLEXOR TENDONS

The volar approach gives the best possible exposure of the flexor tendons within their fibrous sheaths.[17] It also gives excellent exposure of both neurovascular bundles in the finger. The skin incision can be extended into the palm, the volar surface of the wrist, and the anterior surface of the forearm, making it a suitable approach in cases of trauma, where many levels may have to be exposed. Its other major advantage is that many skin lacerations can be incorporated into the skin incision. Its uses include the following:

1. Exploration and repair of flexor tendons
2. Exploration and repair of digital nerves and vessels
3. Exposure of the fibrous flexor sheath for drainage of pus
4. Excision of tumors within the fibrous flexor sheath
5. Excision of palmar fascia in Dupuytren's contracture

POSITION OF PATIENT

Place the patient supine on the operating table with his arm abducted and placed on an arm board. Adjust the height of the table so that you can sit comfortably. Most right-handed surgeons prefer to sit on the ulnar side of the affected arm. An exsanguinating bandage and tourniquet and good lighting are essential (see Fig. 5-13).

LANDMARKS AND INCISION

Landmarks

Three major skin creases traverse the fingers: the *distal phalangeal crease,* just proximal to the distal interphalangeal joint; the *proximal phalangeal crease,* just proximal to the proximal interphalangeal joint; and the *palmar digital crease,* well distal to the metacarpophalangeal joint. The course of the volar zigzag incision takes these creases into account, running diagonally across the finger between creases (Fig. 5-37).

Incision

Before you incise the fingers, mark the skin with methylene blue to outline the proposed site. The angles of the zigzag should be about 90° to each other (or 45° to the transverse skin crease); angles considerably less than 90° to each other may well lead to necrosis of the corners (Fig. 5-38*A*). The angles should not be placed too far dorsally; otherwise, the neuromuscular bundle may be damaged when you mobilize the skin flaps (Fig. 5-38*B*). Of course, the basic zigzag pattern should be modified to accommodate any preexisting lacerations (Fig. 5-39).

INTERNERVOUS PLANE

There is no true internervous plane. The skin flaps are innervated by both the median and the ulnar digital nerves, and no areas of anesthesia are created by the incision.

SUPERFICIAL SURGICAL DISSECTION

Reflect the skin flaps carefully with a skin hook, starting at the apex. Elevate the flaps along with some underlying fat. Do not mobilize the flaps widely until you reach the level of the flexor sheath, to ensure thick flaps and reduce the risk of skin flap necrosis (Fig. 5-40 and *inset*).

DEEP SURGICAL DISSECTION

To expose the flexor tendons, carefully incise the subcutaneous tissues along the midline in a longitudinal fashion (Fig. 5-41). The flexor tendons lie directly underneath, within their fibrous flexor sheaths.

To expose the digital nerve and vessel, gently separate the subcutaneous tissues at the lateral border of the fibrous flexor sheath. The neurovascular bundle is separated from the volar subcutaneous flap by a thin layer of fibrous tissue, Grayson's ligament. This layer must be opened for full exposure of the neurovascular bundle. The

FIG. 5-36A. Kaplan's cardinal line. Used to locate the motor branch of the median nerve to the thenar muscles.

easiest way to pry the tissues apart is to gently open a small pair of closed scissors so that the blades separate the tissues in a longitudinal plane. The blades are actually working along the line of the digital nerve, maximizing exposure of the nerve while minimizing the chances of accidental laceration (Fig. 5-42; see Fig. 5-40).

To expose the bone, create a plane between the edge of the fibrous flexor sheath and the digital nerves and vessels. (In practice, it is seldom necessary to go this deep; surgery on the osseous structures is usually safer through a midlateral or dorsal incision [see Fig. 5-43].)

Incising the fibrous flexor sheath, retracting the tendons, and incising the periosteum from the volar surface of the bone lead to adhesions within the fibrous flexor sheath. It is very important to note that the consequences of this will be the loss of full function of the finger. Therefore, every effort should be made to avoid this at all costs.

DANGERS

Digital nerves and vessels can be damaged if the skin mobilization extends too dorsally.

Skin flaps should not be cut at too acute an angle. Skin sutures should be meticulous to ensure closure. Skin flaps should be thick enough to avoid skin necrosis (see Fig. 5-39).

HOW TO ENLARGE THE APPROACH

Proximal Extension

The zigzag skin incision can be extended onto the palm, eventually joining the curved incision parallel to the thenar crease that is used for exposure of the structures of the palm, volar surface of the wrist, and anterior surface of the forearm. The key to making these incisions is to avoid crossing flexion creases at 90°, thus preventing the development of flexion contractures, and to leave skin flaps with substantial corners (see Fig 5-39).

FIG. 5-37. The relationship of the skin creases to the tendons and joints of the wrist and hand is seen.

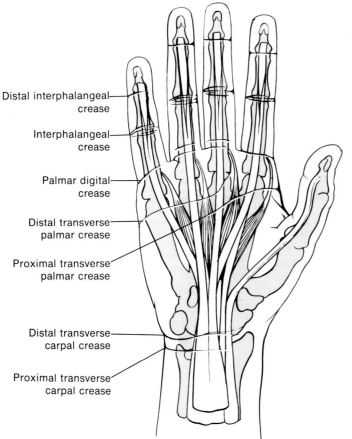

Distal interphalangeal crease

Interphalangeal crease

Palmar digital crease

Distal transverse palmar crease

Proximal transverse palmar crease

Distal transverse carpal crease

Proximal transverse carpal crease

vent the tendons from "bowstringing."

Thickenings in the fibrous flexor sheath are constant (Fig. 5-48). They act as pulleys, directing the sliding movement of the tendons. There are two types: annular and cruciate. Annular pulleys are composed of a single fibrous band (ring); cruciate pulleys have two crossing fibrous strands (cross). Annular pulleys act much like the rings on a fishing rod. Without the ring, the fishing line would pull away from the rod as it bends. This effect is known as bowstringing; in human terms, it results in a loss of range of movement and of power in the affected finger. Annular pulleys include the following:

1. The A1 pulley, which overlies the metacarpophalangeal joint. It is incised during trigger finger release.
2. The A2 pulley, which overlies the proximal end of the proximal phalanx. It must be preserved (if at all possible) to prevent bowstringing.
3. The A3 pulley, which lies over the proximal interphalangeal joint
4. The A4 pulley, which is located about the middle of the middle phalanx. It must be preserved to prevent bowstringing.

Cruciate pulleys, none of which are critical for flexor function, include the following:

1. The C1 pulley, over the middle of the proximal phalanx
2. The C2 pulley, over the proximal end of the middle phalanx
3. The C3 pulley, over the distal end of the middle phalanx

The two tendons enter each fibro-osseous canal with the superficialis tendon on top of the profundus. Over the proximal phalanx, the superficialis tendon divides into halves, which spiral around the profundus tendon, meeting on its deep surface and forming a partial decussation (chiasma). The two then run as one tendon underneath the profundus before attaching to the base of the middle phalanx. Thus, the superficialis tendon actually provides part of the bed on which the profundus tendon runs. Distal to the attachment of the superficialis tendon, the profundus tendon inserts into the base of the terminal phalanx (see Fig. 5-64).

FIG. 5-47. The five zones of the wrist and hand (according to Milford).

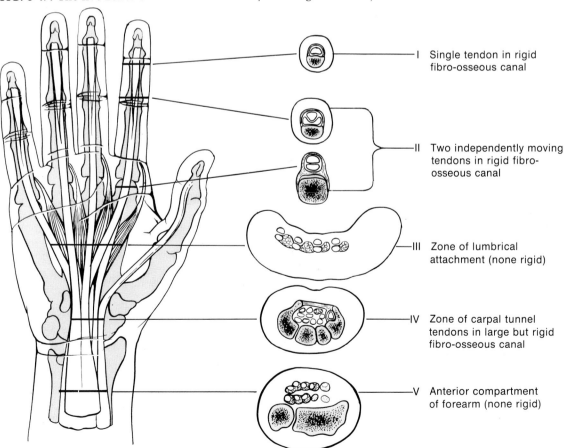

I Single tendon in rigid fibro-osseous canal

II Two independently moving tendons in rigid fibro-osseous canal

III Zone of lumbrical attachment (none rigid)

IV Zone of carpal tunnel tendons in large but rigid fibro-osseous canal

V Anterior compartment of forearm (none rigid)

Within the fibro-osseous sheath, the nutrition of the flexor tendons is provided for by blood vessels that enter the tendons from synovial folds called vincula (Fig. 5-49).

Extremely difficult conditions for full recovery exist after lacerations in zone 2, mainly because the flexor tendons are enclosed within a non-distensible fibro-osseous canal and because, for full function, the tendons must run over each other. It is important to remember that any adhesion between the two can cause malfunction of the finger involved.

This zone gives the worst prognosis of all the zones.[19] It has been nicknamed "no-man's land" by Bunnell.[20]

Zone 1

Zone 1 is the area distal to the insertion of the superficialis tendon. Although the profundus tendon is still tightly enclosed within a fibro-osseous sheath, it runs alone. Therefore, the prognosis for repair of lacerations in this zone is better than that for zone 2, although not as good as for zones 3, 4, and 5.

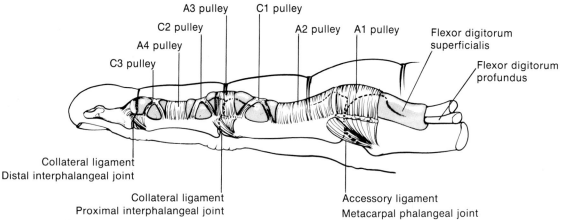

FIG. 5-48. The annular and cruciate ligaments of the flexor tendon sheath, lateral. Note the relationship of the pulleys to the skin creases and joint lines.

FIG. 5-49. The vincula longa and brevia are main blood supplies to the flexor tendons. *(Inset)* Note the relationship of the vincula to the flexor tendon synovial sheath.

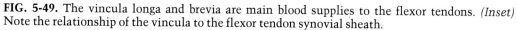

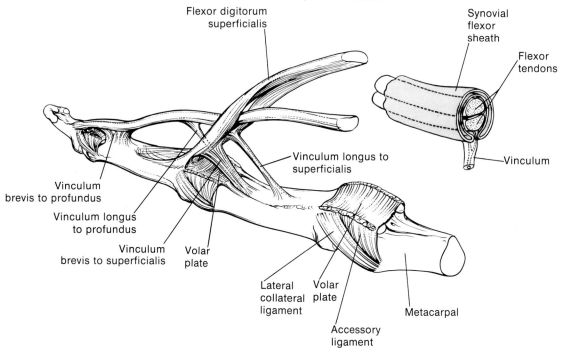

Vascular Supply of the Tendons

Within the fibrous sheath, the flexor tendons are enveloped in a double layer of synovium (Fig. 5-49 *inset*). Each tendon receives its blood supply from arteries that arise from the palmar surface of the phalanges. These vessels are encased in the vinculum (mesotenon). Two vincula supply each tendon, as follows:

A. Profundus tendon
   1. The short vinculum runs to the tendon close to its insertion onto the distal phalanx.
   2. The long vinculum passes to the tendon from between the halves of the superficialis tendon at the level of the proximal phalanx.
B. Superficialis tendon
   1. The short vinculum runs to the tendon near its attachment onto the middle phalanx.
   2. The long vinculum is a double vinculum, passing to each half of the tendon from the palmar surface of the proximal phalanx.

Injection studies on fresh cadaveric material have found that this classic arrangement does not always hold true. The long vincula to both tendons may be absent in the long or ring fingers. When present, the long vinculum to the superficialis may attach to either or both of the slips of the superficialis tendon and the long vinculum to the profundus tendon may arise at the level of the insertion of the superficialis tendon.[21]

These variations should be borne in mind as you explore the flexor tendons within their sheaths.

The vincula should be preserved, if possible, to preserve the blood supply to the tendon.

Other injection studies have found that the volar aspects of the flexor tendons are largely avascular; their nutrition may well be derived from synovial fluid. Therefore, sutures placed in the volar aspect of the tendons do not materially interfere with the blood supply to the tendon itself.[22]

LANDMARKS AND INCISION

The critical landmarks of hand surgery are the skin creases, all situated where the fascia attaches to the skin. There are four major creases: the distal palmar crease corresponds roughly to the palmar location of the metacarpophalangeal joints and the location of the proximal (A1) pulley; the palmar digital crease marks the palmar location of the A2 pulley; the proximal interphalangeal crease marks the proximal interphalangeal joint; and the thenar crease outlines the thenar eminence (see Figs. 5-37, 5-47, and 5-48).

The nerve supply to the skin of the fingers comes from two sources: The volar aspect is supplied by the volar digital nerves; the dorsal aspect is innervated by the dorsal nerves of the radial and ulnar nerves, as well as by the dorsal contribution from the volar digital nerves for the distal 1½ phalanges of the index, long, and ring fingers. The dorsum of the thumb is served exclusively by the radial nerve, and the dorsum of the small finger, by the ulnar nerve. Because of this anatomical arrangement, the midlateral approach to the flexor sheath does not cause skin denervation (see Fig. 5-43).

VOLAR APPROACH TO THE SCAPHOID

The volar approach gives good exposure of the scaphoid bone.[23] It also avoids damaging the dorsal blood supply to the bone's proximal half, as well as the superficial branch of the radial nerve. However, it does pose a threat to the radial artery, which is close to the operative field. It leaves a more cosmetic scar than the dorsal approach. Its uses include the following:

1. Bone grafting for nonunion of the scaphoid
2. Excision of the proximal third of the scaphoid
3. Excision of the radial styloid, either alone or combined with one of the above procedures

POSITION OF PATIENT

Place the patient supine on the operating table, with his arm on an arm board. Supinate the forearm to expose the volar aspect of the wrist, and apply an exsanguinating bandage and tourniquet (see Fig. 5-13).

LANDMARKS AND INCISION

Landmarks

Palpate the *tuberosity of the scaphoid* on the volar

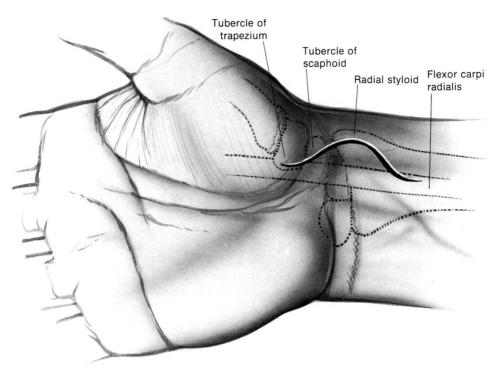

FIG. 5-50. Incision for the volar approach to the scaphoid. Base the incision on the tuberosity of the scaphoid and extend it proximally and distally. The proximal extension is between the tendon of the flexor carpi radialis and the radial artery.

aspect of the wrist, just distal to the skin crease of the wrist joint.

The *flexor carpi radialis* lies radial to the palmaris longus at the level of the wrist. It crosses the scaphoid before inserting into the base of the second and third metacarpal just on the ulnar side of the radial pulse.

Incision

Make a vertical or curvilinear incision on the volar aspect of the wrist, some 2 cm to 3 cm long. Base it on the tuberosity of the scaphoid and extend it proximally between the tendon of the flexor carpi radialis and the radial artery (Fig. 5-50).

INTERNERVOUS PLANE

There is no true internervous plane; the only muscle mobilized is the flexor carpi radialis (median nerve).

SUPERFICIAL SURGICAL DISSECTION

Incise the deep fascia in line with the skin incision and identify the radial artery on the lateral (radial) side of the wound (Fig. 5-51). Retract the radial artery and lateral skin flap to the lateral side. Identify the tendon of the flexor carpi radialis and then retract the tendon medially to expose the volar aspect of the radial side of the wrist joint (Fig. 5-52).

DEEP SURGICAL DISSECTION

Incise the capsule of the wrist joint over the scaphoid to expose the distal two thirds of the scaphoid. This anterior area of bone is nonarticular. To gain the best view of the proximal third of the bone, dorsiflex the wrist markedly (Fig. 5-53).

DANGERS

Vessels

The **radial artery** lies close to the lateral border of the wound and can be accidentally incised at any time during the dissection. It must be identified early in the dissection.

Note that this approach exposes the distal two thirds of the scaphoid.

HOW TO ENLARGE THE APPROACH

The incision can be usefully extended to a limited extent. By carrying it proximally, fracture of the distal radius can be approached. Also, this is adequate exposure to allow you to take a bone graft from the radial styloid or the volar aspect of the radius. Most nonunions occur in the proximal third of the scaphoid and may be difficult to find unless you dorsiflex the wrist. If you are not completely certain about where the fracture is, place a small radiopaque marker at the operative site and carry out a radiographic examination on the table.

182

DRAINAGE OF THE LATERAL (THENAR) SPACE

INCISION

Make a curved incision about 4 cm long, just on the ulnar side of the thenar crease (Fig. 5-71).

INTERNERVOUS PLANE

There is no internervous plane.

SUPERFICIAL SURGICAL DISSECTION

Deepen the dissection in line with the skin incision, taking care to identify and preserve the digital nerves to the index finger. Identify the long flexor tendon to the index finger (Figs. 5-72 and 5-73). Deep to these tendons is the lateral space; enter it by blunt dissection (Fig. 5-74).

DANGERS

Nerves

The **digital nerves** to the index finger are directly in line with the skin incision. Take care not to damage them when you incise the palmar aponeurosis.

The **motor branch to the thenar muscles** emerges from the deep surface of the median nerve as the median nerve leaves the carpal tunnel. Note, however, that the location of its division from the median nerve is quite variable. This nerve hooks around the distal end of the flexor retinaculum to supply the muscles. Make sure you identify the branch at the proximal end of the incision so that you do not damage it (see Fig. 5-32).

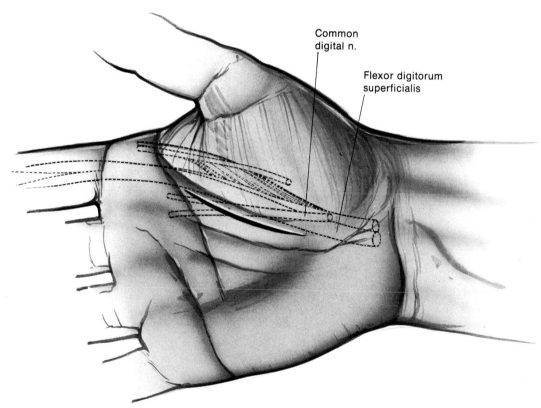

Common
digital n.

Flexor digitorum
superficialis

FIG. 5-71. Incision for the drainage of the lateral space (thenar space). The incision is made just to the ulnar side of the thenar crease.

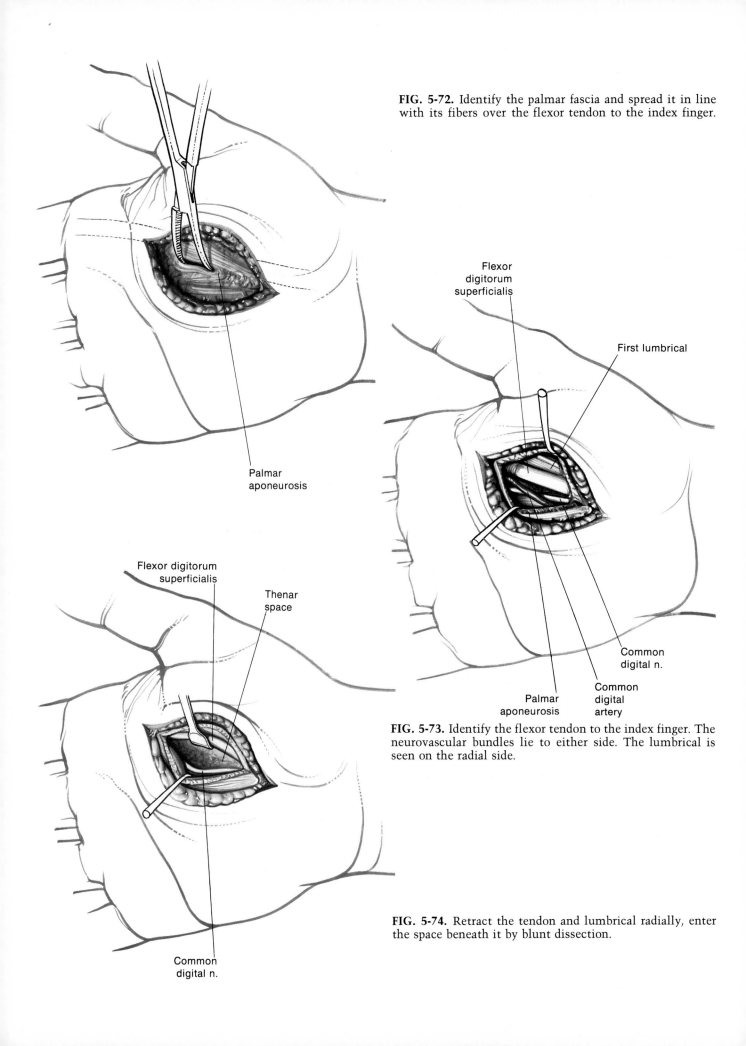

FIG. 5-72. Identify the palmar fascia and spread it in line with its fibers over the flexor tendon to the index finger.

Palmar
aponeurosis

Flexor
digitorum
superficialis

First lumbrical

Common
digital n.

Common
digital
artery

Palmar
aponeurosis

FIG. 5-73. Identify the flexor tendon to the index finger. The neurovascular bundles lie to either side. The lumbrical is seen on the radial side.

Flexor digitorum
superficialis

Thenar
space

Common
digital n.

FIG. 5-74. Retract the tendon and lumbrical radially, enter the space beneath it by blunt dissection.

APPLIED SURGICAL ANATOMY OF THE DEEP PALMAR SPACE

The palm is divided into spaces by fibrous septa that pass through it before attaching to the metacarpals. There are two major septa: The *thenar septum* originates from the palmar aponeurosis and inserts into the first metacarpal, separating the three muscles of the thenar eminence from the central palmar structures; the *hypothenar septum* originates on the ulnar side of the palmar aponeurosis and inserts into the fifth metacarpal, separating the three muscles of the hypothenar eminence from the central palmar structures (see Figs. 5-34 and 5-66).

The palm is thus divided into three compartments: a thenar compartment, a hypothenar compartment, and a central compartment.

The central compartment contains the long flexor tendons to the fingers and the adductor pollicis, as well as the digital nerves and vessels and the superficial and deep palmar arches.

Within the central compartment, a *potential deep space* exists between the undersurface of the flexor tendons and the upper surface of the interossei and adductor pollicis. This deep palmar space is divided into medial (midpalmar) and lateral (thenar) spaces by the *oblique septum* that arises from the connective tissue surrounding the middle finger flexor tendons and runs to the palmar surface of the middle metacarpal.[26] This septum is the anatomical basis for the clinical division of deep palmar infection into two distinct separate spaces.[25]

LATERAL SPACE (THENAR SPACE)

The lateral space usually contains the first lumbrical muscle, which runs with the long flexor tendon to the index finger. Infections in the first web space may track down into the lateral space along the lumbrical, although this is rare. While lateral space infections may be drained through the first web space, such an incision drains less thoroughly than the procedure described in the previous section (see Figs. 5-71 through 5-74).

The space lies anterior to the adductor pollicis muscle. A second potential space exists behind that muscle and in front of the interossei. Infection of this "posterior adductor space" is very rare indeed.[27]

MEDIAL SPACE (MIDPALMAR SPACE)

The medial space contains the lumbricals for the middle, ring, and little fingers, which run from the long flexor tendons of the middle, ring, and little fingers (the volar boundary of the space). The deep boundary is formed by the interossei and metacarpals of the third and fourth spaces. Thus, infection in the web spaces between the middle and ring fingers and between the ring and little fingers may in theory spread to the medial space (see Fig. 5-66). The medial space may be drained through an incision in these webs, but the result is not as good as direct drainage (see Figs. 5-67 through 5-70).

DRAINAGE OF THE RADIAL BURSA

The long flexor tendon of the thumb is surrounded by a synovial sheath that extends from the tendon's insertion into the distal phalanx through the palm and carpal tunnel to the forearm just proximal to the proximal end of the flexor retinaculum. The proximal end of this sheath is known as the radial bursa (Fig. 5-75).

Infection of this space is diagnosed on the same clinical grounds as infections of the synovial sheaths of the other fingers: fusiform swelling of the thumb, with extreme pain on active or passive extension of the digit.

POSITION OF PATIENT

Place the patient supine on the operating table, with his arm on an arm board. A general anesthetic or an axillary or brachial block is essential. Use a

nonexsanguinating tourniquet and have an excellent light source available (see Fig. 5-12).

LANDMARKS AND INCISION

Landmark

The *interphalangeal crease of the thumb* is the surface marking for the interphalangeal joint of the thumb. It lies just proximal to the distal end of the fibrous flexor sheath of the thumb.

Incision

Two incisions are required for complete drainage: First, make a small longitudinal incision on the lateral side of the proximal phalanx of the thumb, just dorsal to the dorsal termination of the interphalangeal crease (Fig. 5-76). Then make a second incision over the medial aspect of the thenar emi-

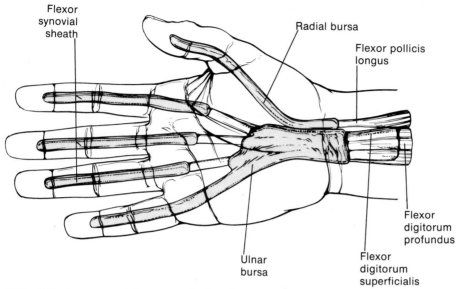

FIG. 5-75. Anatomy of the synovial sheaths of the fingers and the radial and ulnar bursae.

FIG. 5-76. Incision for drainage of the radial bursa. Two incisions are required for complete drainage. Distally, make a small longitudinal incision on the lateral side of the proximal phalanx of the thumb, just dorsal to the interphalangeal crease. Make a second incision over the medial aspect of the thenar eminence on the volar aspect of the wrist, and carry the incision proximally to the end of the radial bursa. Care must be taken to protect the median nerve and its motor branch to the thenar muscles.

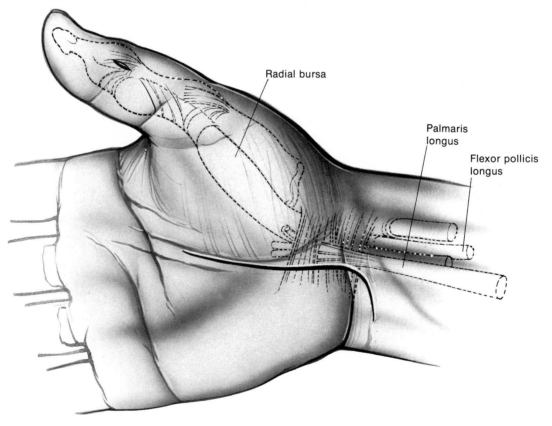

FIG. 6-7.

(**A**) Insert a blunt dissector under the cut edge of the ligamentum flavum.

(**B**) Use a Kerrison Leskel to remove the distal end of the lamina. Note that the ligamentum flavum attaches halfway up the undersurface of the lamina.

(**C**) Remove additional lamina and the remaining portion of the ligamentum flavum at its attachment to the undersurface of the lamina.

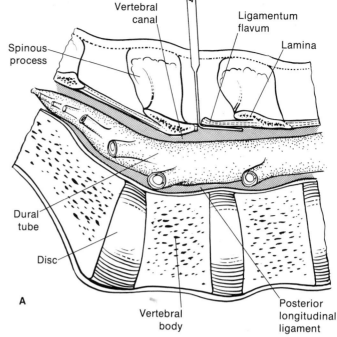

A

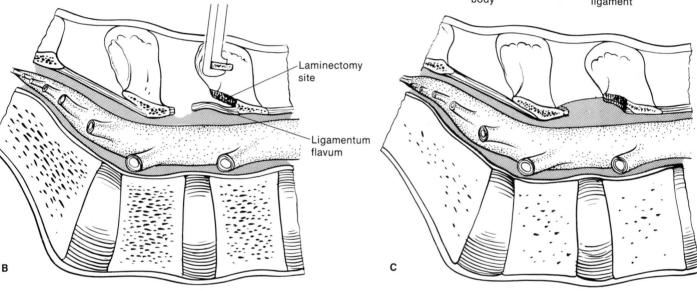

B

C

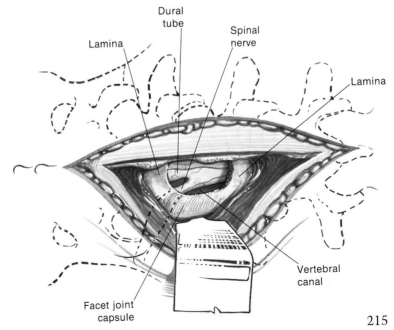

FIG. 6-8. Immediately beneath the ligamentum flavum and epidural fat is the blue white dura. Identify the nerve root. Note the overlying epidural veins.

215

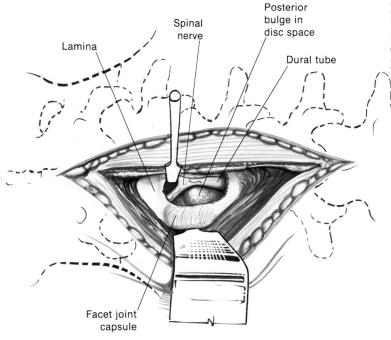

FIG. 6-9. Using blunt dissection, carefully continue down the lateral side of the dura to the floor of the spinal canal; retract the dura and its nerve root medially. Reveal the posterior aspect of the disc space.

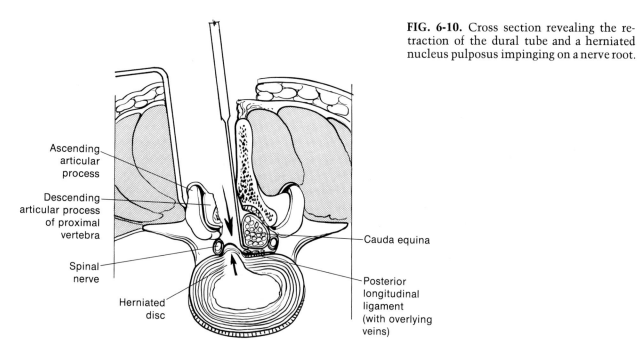

FIG. 6-10. Cross section revealing the retraction of the dural tube and a herniated nucleus pulposus impinging on a nerve root.

2. To gain access to other parts of the posterior aspect of the spine, carry the dissection as far laterally as possible, onto the transverse processes. Complete lateral dissection exposes the facet joints and transverse processes, permitting facet joint fusion and transverse process fusion, if necessary (see Fig. 6-5).

Extensile Measures

To extend the approach, merely extend the skin incision proximally or distally and detach the posterior spinal musculature from the posterior spinal elements. The approach is extensile from C1 down to the sacrum.

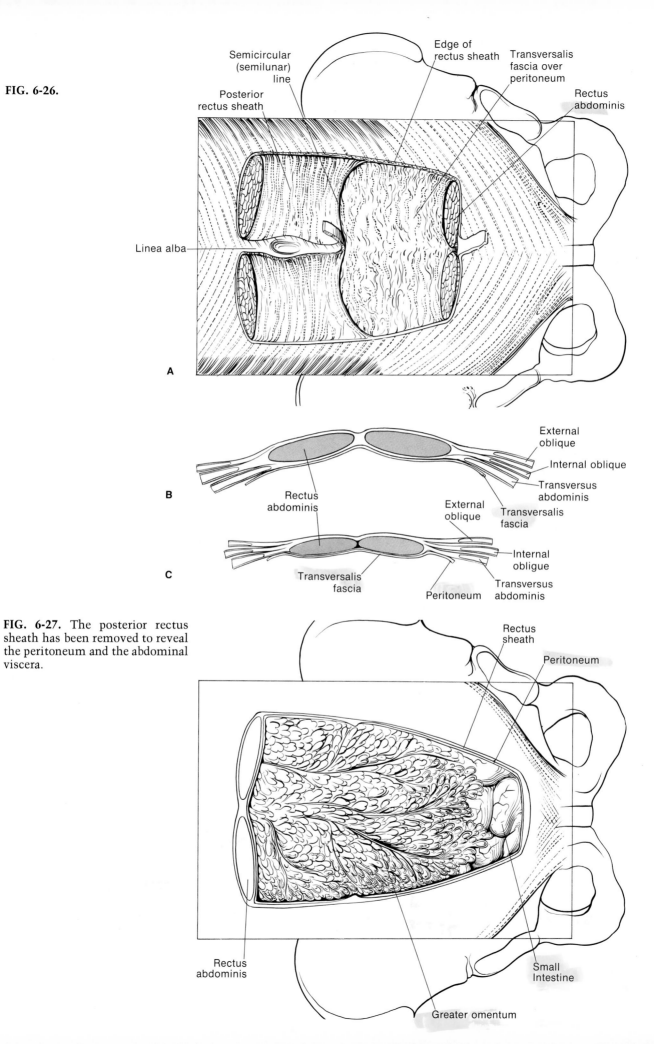

FIG. 6-26.

Semicircular (semilunar) line

Posterior rectus sheath

Edge of rectus sheath

Transversalis fascia over peritoneum

Rectus abdominis

Linea alba

A

B

Rectus abdominis

External oblique

Internal oblique

Transversus abdominis

Transversalis fascia

External oblique

Transversalis fascia

Internal oblique

Transversus abdominis

C

Peritoneum

FIG. 6-27. The posterior rectus sheath has been removed to reveal the peritoneum and the abdominal viscera.

Rectus sheath

Peritoneum

Rectus abdominis

Greater omentum

Small Intestine

DEEP SURGICAL DISSECTION AND ITS DANGERS

The deep surgical dissection consists of freeing the distal ends of the aorta and the vena cava from the vertebrae in the L4–L5 vertebral area. The aorta divides on the anterior surface of the L4 vertebra into the two common iliac arteries. Just below this bifurcation, the common iliac vessels divide in turn at approximately the S1 level into the internal and external iliac vessels. The internal iliac is the more medial of the two (Fig. 6-28).

The aorta and vena cava are held firmly onto the anterior parts of the lower lumbar vertebrae by the lumbar vessels. These segmental vessels must be mobilized to permit the aorta and vena cava to be moved (see Fig. 6-14). Because arterial structures are easier to dissect and more muscular than the thin-walled venous structures, the preferred approach to the L4–L5 disc is from the left, the more arterial side. The median sacral artery originates from the aorta at its bifurcation at L4 and runs in the midline, over the sacral promontory and down into the hollow of the sacrum (see Fig. 6-28). The lumbosacral disc usually lies in the V formed by the two common iliac vessels. Nevertheless, the level at which the vessels bifurcate may vary; on rare occasions, they may have to be mobilized to expose the L5–S1 disc.

Note that the left common iliac vein lies below the left common iliac artery, whereas the right common iliac artery lies below and medial to the

FIG. 6-28. The abdominal viscera has been retracted proximally and the retroperitoneum has been resected to reveal the great vessels at their bifurcation, the ureters, and the presacral parasympathetic plexus.

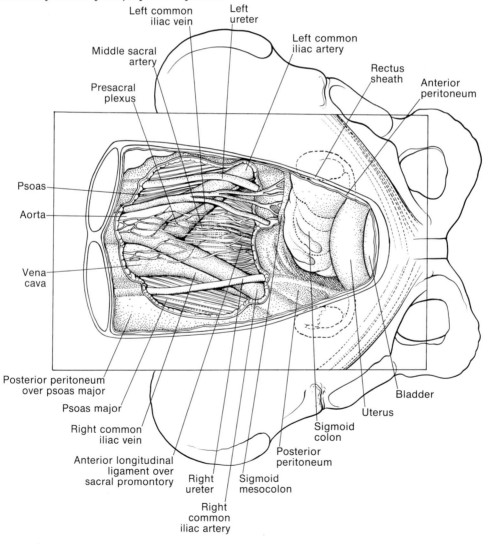

right common iliac vein. Therefore, special care must be taken when mobilizing the left side of the vascular V, since the vessel closest to the surgery is the thin-walled vein, not the artery (Fig. 6-29; see Fig. 6-28).

The parasympathetic nerves in the presacral area exist as a diffuse plexus of nerves running around the aorta, heading inferiorly from the bifurcation and running along the anterior surface of the sacrum beneath the posterior peritoneum. They should be protected, if at all possible, to preserve adequate sexual function and prevent retroejacula-

tion in men. Because of the function of these nerves, this approach is perhaps safer in women than in men (see Figs. 6-28 and 6-29).

The ureter runs down the posterior abdominal wall on the psoas muscle. At the bifurcation of the common iliac artery over the sacroiliac joint, it clings to the posterior abdominal wall, held there by the peritoneum, and should be well lateral to the approach to the L5–S1 disc. It may have to be mobilized for exposure of the L4–L5 disc (Fig. 6-30; see Fig. 6-29).

FIG. 6-29. Portions of the major vessels have been resected to reveal the underlying L5–S1 disc space, the sacral promontory, and its overlying presacral plexus.

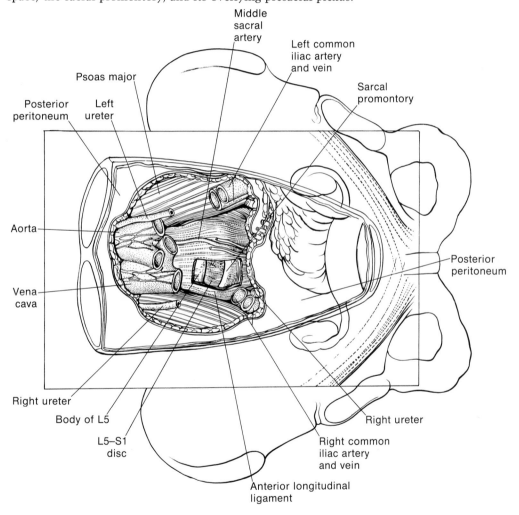

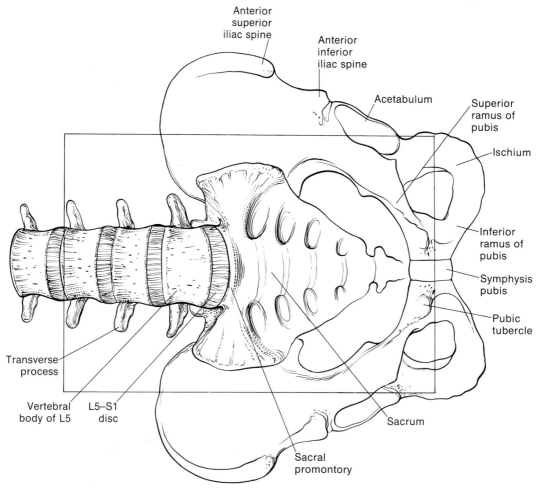

FIG. 6-30. Osteology of the anterior aspect of the pelvis and lumbosacral spine.

ANTEROLATERAL (RETROPERITONEAL) APPROACH TO THE LUMBAR SPINE

The retroperitoneal approach to the anterior part of the lumbar spine has several advantages over the transperitoneal approach. First, it provides access to all vertebrae from L1 to the sacrum, while the transperitoneal approach is difficult to use above the level of L4. Second, it allows drainage of infection, such as a psoas abscess, without the risk of a postoperative ileitis. Because of the arrangement of the vascular anatomy of the retroperitoneal space, however, the approach is slightly more difficult than the transperitoneal approach for reaching the L5–S1 disc space.

The uses of the approach include the following:

1. Spinal fusion
2. Drainage of psoas abscess and curettage of infected vertebral body
3. Resection of all or part of a vertebral body and associated bone grafting
4. Biopsy of a vertebral body when a needle biopsy is either not possible or hazardous

The most common use is in general surgery, for exposure of the sympathetic chain.[9]

POSITION OF PATIENT

Place the patient on the operating table in the semilateral position. The patient's body should be at approximately a 45° angle to the horizontal, facing away from you. Keep the patient in this position throughout the surgery by placing sandbags under the hips and shoulders or by using a kidney rest brace to hold the patient. The angle allows the peritoneal contents to fall away from the incision. Alternatively, place the patient supine on the operating table and tilt the table at 45° to the horizontal away from you. This position has the advantage of not putting the psoas muscle on stretch (Fig. 6-31).

For most procedures, have the left side up so that you approach the "aortic" rather than the "caval" side.

LANDMARKS AND INCISION

Landmarks

Palpate the *twelfth rib* in the affected flank and the *pubic symphysis* in the lower part of the abdomen. Palpate the lateral border of the *rectus abdominis muscle* about 5 cm lateral to the midline.

Incision

Make an oblique flank incision extending down from the posterior half of the twelfth rib toward the rectus abdominis muscle and stopping at its lateral border, approximately midway between the umbilicus and the pubic symphysis (Fig. 6-33).

INTERNERVOUS PLANE

No internervous plane is available for use. The three muscles of the abdominal wall (the external oblique, the internal oblique, and the transversus abdominis) are divided in line with the skin incision. Because all three muscles are segmentally innervated, significant denervation does not occur (Fig. 6-32).

SUPERFICIAL SURGICAL DISSECTION

Deepen the incision through subcutaneous fat to expose the aponeurosis of the external oblique. Divide the aponeurosis of the external oblique in the line of its fibers, which is in line with the skin incision. The muscle fibers of the external oblique rarely appear below the level of the umbilicus except in very muscular patients. If you find them, split the muscle in the line of its fibers (Fig. 6-34).

Next, divide the internal oblique in line with the skin incision and perpendicular to the line of its muscular fibers. This division causes partial denervation, but if the muscle is closed properly, post-

FIG. 6-31. Place the patient in the semilateral position for the anterolateral (retroperitoneal) approach to the lumbar spine.

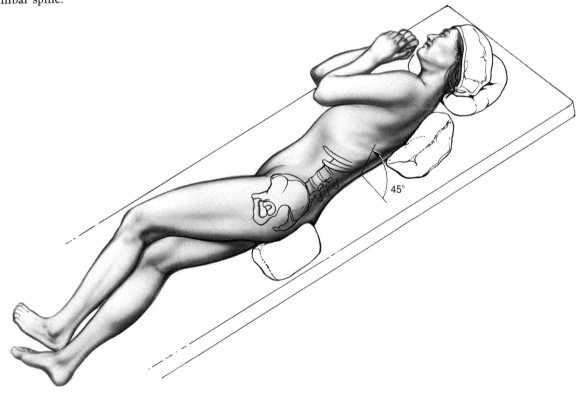

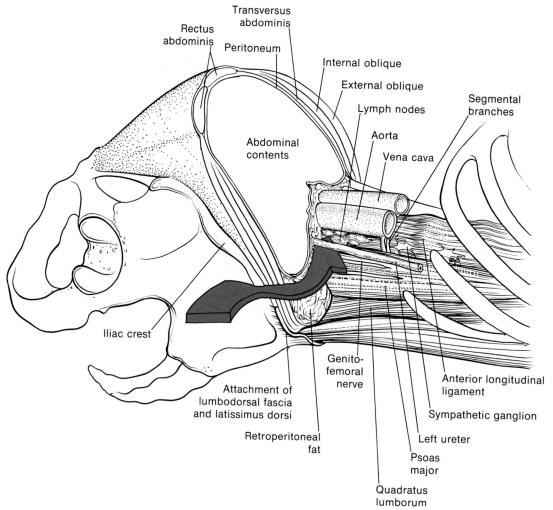

FIG. 6-32. The anterior abdominal musculature and viscera have been transected and removed at the level of the iliac crest. The arrow indicates the route of surgery between the peritoneum anteriorly and the retroperitoneal structures posteriorly.

operative hernias can be avoided (Fig. 6-35). Under the internal oblique lies the transversus abdominis. It, too, should be divided in line with the skin incision to expose the retroperitoneal space (Figs. 6-36, 6-37, 6-41, and 6-42).

Using blunt finger dissection, develop a plane between the retroperitoneal fat and the fascia that lies over the psoas muscle (Fig. 6-38). Gently mobilize the peritoneal cavity and its contents and retract them medially (Fig. 6-39). Carry out this dissection from either the left lower quadrant or the right upper quadrant, depending on the side you wish to expose.

Because the aorta is on the left, the exposure used for routine spinal fusion comes from the left side. Place a Dever retractor over the peritoneal contents and retract them to the right upper quadrant. The ureter, which is loosely attached to the peritoneum, is carried forward with it.

DEEP SURGICAL DISSECTION

Identify the psoas fascia, but do not enter the muscle. Any existing psoas abscess is easily palpable at this point. If you find one, enter it from its lateral side with finger dissection. Follow the abscess cavity with your finger directly to the infected disc space or spaces. If there is no psoas abscess, follow the surface of the psoas muscle medially to reach the anterior lateral surface of the vertebral bodies.

The aorta and vena cava are effectively tied to the waist of the vertebral bodies by the lumbar arteries and veins. These smaller vessels must be individually located on the vertebrae involved and tied so that you can mobilize the aorta and vena cava and reach the anterior part of the vertebral body. Make sure that the lumbar vessels are not cut flush with the aorta; a slipped tie would then

APPLIED SURGICAL ANATOMY OF THE ANTERIOR APPROACH TO THE CERVICAL SPINE

OVERVIEW

The key to understanding the anatomy of the approach lies in the appreciation of the three fascial layers of the neck. The most superficial fascial layer is the investing layer of *deep cervical fascia*. The fascia surrounds the neck like a collar but splits around the sternocleidomastoid and trapezius muscles to enclose them. Posteriorly, it joins with the ligamentum nuchae (nuchal ligament). The superficial layer is incised along the anterior border of the sternocleidomastoid. Dividing the fascia layer allows the sternocleidomastoid to be retracted laterally and to be separated from the underlying strap muscles. The only structures superficial to it are the platysma (a remnant of the old panniculus carnosus, or muscle of the skin) and the external jugular vein, which can be divided safely if it intrudes into the operative field (Figs. 6-71 and 6-72).

The next fascial layer is the *pretracheal fascia*, which forms a layer between sliding surfaces. It invests the strap muscles and runs from the hyoid bone down into the chest (see Fig. 6-72). Its key relationship is with the carotid sheath, which encloses the common carotid artery, the internal jugular vein, and the vagus nerve. The pretracheal

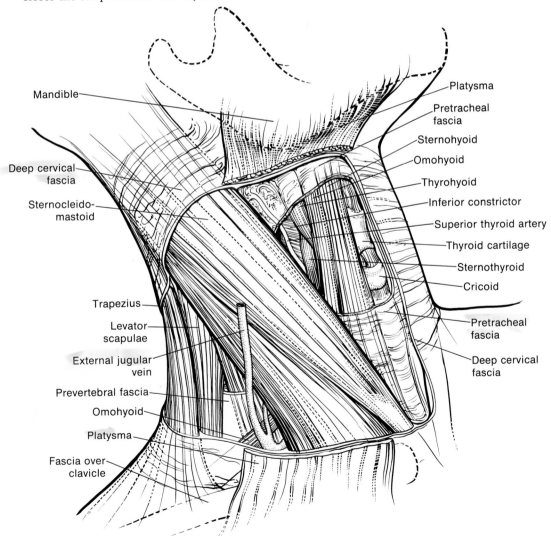

FIG. 6-72. The platysma and deep cervical fascia have been removed. Note that the deep cervical fascia (investing fascia) encloses the sternocleidomastoid. The deeper pretracheal fascia encloses the strap muscles and thyroid structures.

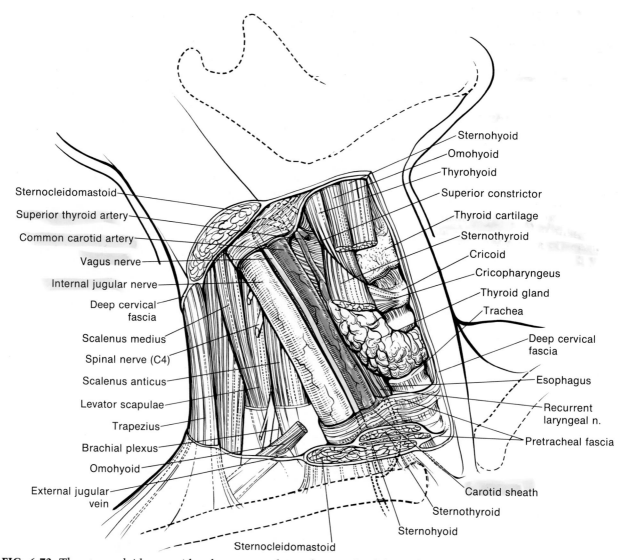

FIG. 6-73. The sternocleidomastoid and strap muscles and pretracheal fascia have been resected. The carotid sheath and its contents have been exposed. The thyroid gland, cartilage, and trachea are seen. Note the course of the recurrent laryngeal nerve.

fascia is continuous with the carotid sheath at the sheath's lateral margin (see Figs. 6-71 and 6-73). Hence, the pretracheal fascia must be divided on the medial border of the carotid sheath so that the carotid sheath can be retracted laterally and the midline structures medially. Two sets of vessels, the superior and inferior thyroid vessels, run from the carotid sheath through the pretracheal fascia into the midline. On rare occasions, the thyroid vessels have to be divided to enlarge the exposure (see Fig. 6-74). However, the superior laryngeal nerve, which runs with the superior thyroid vessels, must be preserved.

The deepest layer of fascia is the *prevertebral fascia,* a firm, tough membrane that lies in front of the prevertebral muscles. On its surface runs the cervical sympathetic trunk, which lies roughly over the transverse processes of the cervical vertebrae. Beneath the prevertebral fascia are the left and right longus colli muscles (see Figs. 6-71 and 6-74).

LANDMARKS AND INCISION

Landmarks

The *carotid tubercle* is the enlargement of the anterior tubercle of the transverse process of C6. It is larger than all other vertebral tubercles (there is no anterior tubercle of C7) and may be palpable. The tubercle of C6 is the key surgical landmark in the anterior incision (see Fig. 6-76).

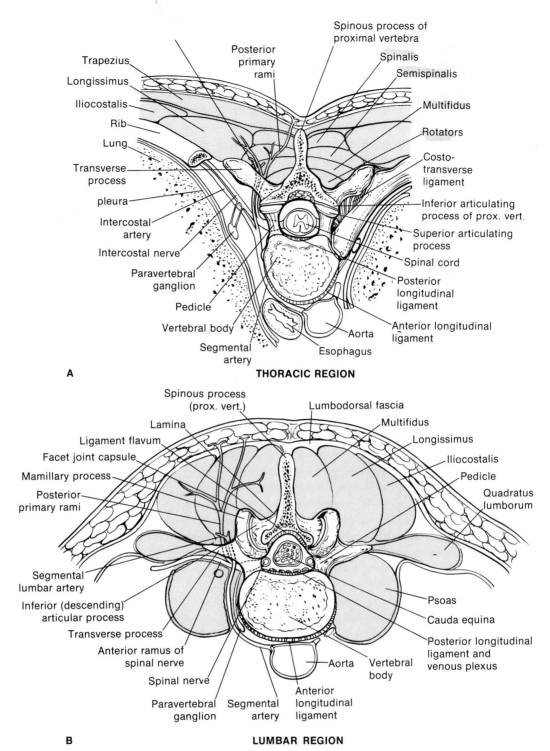

FIG. 6-105 (A) Cross section through the level of a thoracic vertebra. Superficial and deep layers of the thoracic spine are visualized, as well as their nerve and blood supply. **(B)** Cross section through the level of a lumbar vertebra. Note that the individual muscles of the sacrospinalis musculature are one paravertebral mass at this level. Note that the medial end of the cup-shaped ascending articulating process is closest to the lumbar nerve root.

layer of epidural fat. The dura must be protected; any epidural tear must be closed off (see Figs. 6-12 and 6-13).

The cup-shaped ascending articulating process is closest to the lumbar nerve root. Arthritis of the medial end of the ascending facet can cause compression of the nerve in the foramen. The nerve root is safe during the foramenotomy if the anatomical arrangement of the facet joints to the nerve root is appreciated. Protect the nerve root during the removal of the medial portion of the ascending process, the portion that is close to the nerve root (see Fig. 6-105B).

291

APPROACH TO THE POSTERIOR LATERAL THORAX FOR EXCISION OF RIBS

After you have completed scoliosis surgery, you may have to resect portions of the ribs on the posterolateral aspect of the rib cage to flatten out a hump caused by ribs that still protrude.

POSITION OF PATIENT

Place the patient prone on the operating table. Position bolsters longitudinally on either side of the patient from the anterior superior iliac spine to the shoulders to allow room for chest expansion (see Fig. 6-95).

LANDMARKS AND INCISION

Landmarks

The best landmarks are the *prominent ribs,* usually on the right posterior thoracic region. They may be so distorted that they produce a "razorback" deformity.

Incision

The standard incision for scoliosis surgery, the longitudinal midline incision, is also used for the removal of ribs (see Fig. 6-96).

INTERNERVOUS PLANE

The internervous plane lies between the trapezius and the latissimus dorsi. The trapezius is innervated by the spinal accessory nerve, and the latissimus dorsi is innervated by the long thoracic (thoracodorsal) nerve. The deeper muscle, the iliocostalis portion of the sacrospinalis, is segmentally innervated and is therefore not denervated when split longitudinally.

SUPERFICIAL SURGICAL DISSECTION

With retractors, lift the skin and its thick subcutaneous tissue. Free them from the underlying fascia and retract them laterally. Center the dissection over the most prominent, or apical, rib; extend it laterally to at least 12 cm from the midline and proximally and distally to expose all the deformed ribs (Fig. 6-106).

INTERMEDIATE SURGICAL DISSECTION

The trapezius fibers run obliquely downward toward the midline as far as the spinous process of T12. Identify it by its rolled, lateral free border. Dissect along the lateral border and retract the muscle medially. The medial portion of the latissimus dorsi's fibers and the aponeurosis run almost perpendicular to and under the trapezius; it takes origin from the lower six thoracic spinous processes as well as from the lumbodorsal fascia. Dissect the muscle free with a cautery and retract it laterally (see Fig. 6-106).

DEEP SURGICAL DISSECTION

Below the retracted trapezius and latissimus dorsi lies the iliocostalis, a longitudinal muscle with flattened tendons in its musculature that insert into the lower borders of the ribs. Split the iliocostalis longitudinally over each of the deformed portions of the ribs you are removing and then dissect and retract it medially and laterally in line with the ribs (Fig. 6-107).

Incise the periosteum along the posterior aspect of the rib in the rib's own plane. Use an Alexander dissector to push the split periosteum to the upper and lower borders of the rib. With the special end of the dissector, strip the intercostal muscles off the upper end of the rib from medial to lateral in the angle formed by the intersection of the external intercostals and the rib. Then strip the intercostals from the lower end of the rib from lateral to medial, remaining in the angle formed by the origin of the external intercostal and the rib to discourage bleeding. By keeping your dissection subperiosteal, you avoid the neurovascular bundle, which will have been freed from the lower border of the rib with the intercostal muscles (Fig. 6-108).

Before continuing, have the anesthesiologist stop the patient from breathing so that the viseral pleura can fall away from the rib, minimizing the danger to the pleura as you dissect anteriorly. When you have completely uncovered the ribs, begin to resect them.

DANGERS

The **neurovascular bundle** lies along the lower edge of the rib in the neurovascular groove. Unless you keep the dissection subperiosteal, you may inadvertently cut it during the resection and be forced to cauterize the intercostal vessels, causing possible segmental chest wall numbness (see Fig. 108 *inset*).

Violating the pleura may result in a **pneumothorax.** If that happens, plan to insert a chest tube immediately after you close the wound, while you are still in the operating room.

Connecting the midline wound with that of the

rib resection may cause a **hemothorax,** with blood flowing from the area of the spinal fusion into the lung. If you do connect the two areas of dissection, be prepared to insert a chest tube to drain the blood.

The **skin** may adhere to the cut ends of the ribs, causing unsightly dimpling. To prevent it, take a thick subcutaneous layer with the skin and during closure suture the fascia of the trapezius to that of the latissimus dorsi.

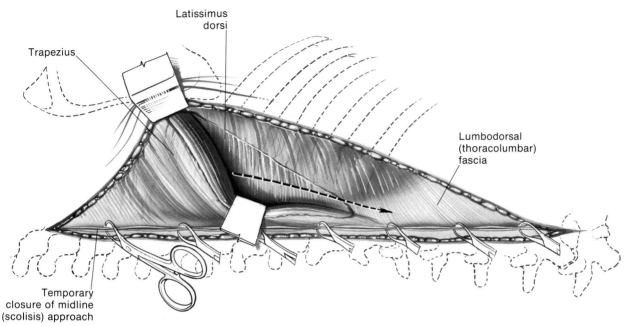

FIG. 6-106. Retract the rolled lateral border of the trapezius muscle medially to expose the thin, aponeurotic medial portion of the latissimus dorsi. Incise the aponeurotic medial portion of the latissimus dorsi perpendicular to its fibers.

FIG. 6-107. Retract the latissimus dorsi laterally and the trapezius medially to expose the underlying iliocostalis muscle. Incise the muscle longitudinally, parallel to its fibers.

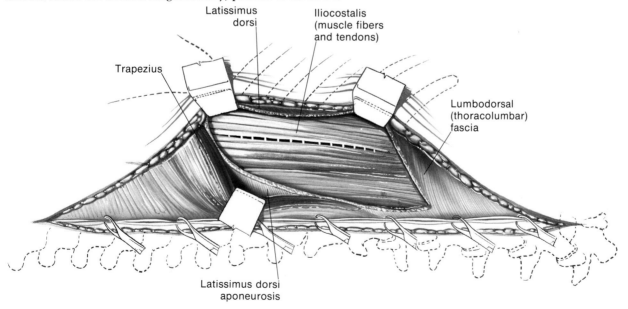

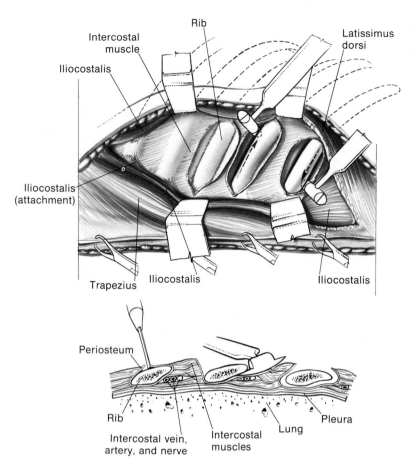

FIG. 6-108. Dissect and retract the iliocostalis muscles laterally and medially from their insertion to expose the posterior aspect of the ribs. Incise the periosteum over the rib. Push the split periosteum to the upper and lower borders of the rib. With a special dissector, strip the intercostal muscles off the borders of the rib as well as anteriorly.

HOW TO ENLARGE THE APPROACH

Local Measures

Continue subcutaneous dissection further laterally, proximally, and distally to ensure a complete view of the distorted ribs.

Occasionally, in more proximal rib resections, you may have to dissect the lower portion of the rhomboid major to expose the rib area more fully. Distally, you may have to split the muscular belly of the iliocostalis, as it splits from the sacrospinalis.

Extensile Measures

The incision is not extensile; deciding which ribs to remove depends on the size and extent of the rib hump.

SPECIAL POINTS

When removing ribs, resect each one from the point just lateral to its maximum deformity to the most medial end, without removing its head and neck. The lateral portion of the resected rib will drop forward, reducing the rib hump, but the medial portion, held rigidly in place by the costotransverse ligament and the costovertebral ligament, will not move. That is why you should resect the rib as medially as possible. Otherwise, the medial end of the rib will continue to stick out posteriorly, causing continued deformity.

Removing more than four ribs may cause a sympathetic effusion of a lung field. If a significant effusion occurs, insert a chest tube to drain the fluid.

Treat the cut ends of the ribs with bone wax to prevent continued oozing of blood. The wax does not prevent the ribs from regenerating.

The resected portions of the ribs can be cut into small, matchstick-sized pieces and used as graft material in a midline spine fusion.

If the vertebral body has rotated up under the rib, resecting the ribs will not produce a significant decrease in the rib hump deformity.

POSTERIOR APPROACH TO THE ILIAC CREST FOR BONE GRAFT

Posterior iliac crest bone grafts are usually taken during any posterior spine surgery that requires additional autogenous bone to supplement the area to be fused. The grafts may also be used as cortical cancellous grafts for any part of the skeleton that needs fusion or refusion.

POSITION OF PATIENT

Place the patient prone on the operating table, with bolsters running longitudinally to support the chest wall and pelvis, allowing the chest wall and abdomen to expand without touching the table. Place drapes distally enough so that you can see the beginning of the gluteal cleft and the posterior superior iliac spines (see Fig. 6-95).

LANDMARKS AND INCISION

Landmarks

Palpate the *posterior superior iliac spine* under the dimpling of the skin above the buttock. The subcutaneous iliac crest is also palpable.

Incision

Make an 8-cm oblique incision, centered over the posterior superior iliac spine and in line with the iliac crest (Fig. 6-109 *inset*).

If you are performing scoliosis surgery or lumbar surgery, you can extend the midline incision distally to the sacrum. Then retract the skin and a thick fatty subcutaneous layer laterally. Using a Hibbs retractor, dissect the flap free from the underlying lumbodorsal fascia until you can palpate and see the posterior superior iliac spine and crest (Fig. 6-109).

INTERNERVOUS PLANE

Muscles insert or take origin from the iliac crest but do not cross it. Therefore, the outer border of the iliac crest is truly an internervous plane. The gluteus medius, minimus, and maximus take their origins from the outer surface of the ilium (the gluteus medius and minimus are supplied by the superior gluteal nerve and the gluteus maximus by the inferior gluteal nerve). The segmentally sup-

FIG. 6-109. If you are performing lumbar spine surgery, extend the midline incision distally, retracting the skin laterally until you can palpate and see the posterior superior iliac spine and crest. Incise the soft tissues overlying the crest down to bone. *(Inset)* Make an 8-cm oblique incision, centered over the posterior superior iliac spine and in line with the iliac crest.

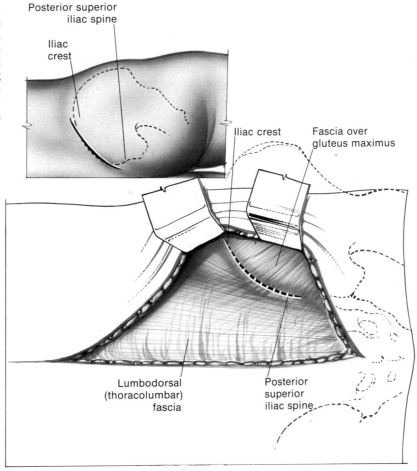

Posterior superior iliac spine

Iliac crest

Iliac crest

Fascia over gluteus maximus

Lumbodorsal (thoracolumbar) fascia

Posterior superior iliac spine

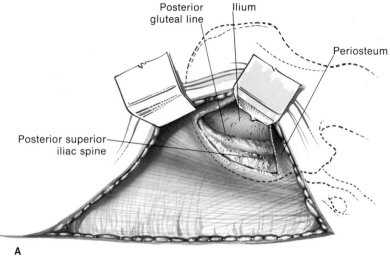

Posterior gluteal line

Ilium

Periosteum

Posterior superior iliac spine

A

FIG. 6-110.

(A) Subperiosteally, strip the musculature off the posterior portion of the lateral surface of the ilium.

(B) As you proceed down the outer surface of the ilium in the area of the posterior superior spine, you will see and feel the elevated posterior gluteal line; pass subperiosteally up and over the line and then down its other side. Do not err by letting the line direct you outward from bone to muscle. If you draw an imaginary line from the posterior superior iliac spine perpendicular to the operating table and stay cephalad to it, you will avoid the sciatic notch and its contents.

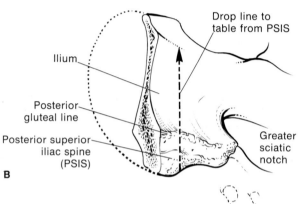

Drop line to table from PSIS

Ilium

Posterior gluteal line

Posterior superior iliac spine (PSIS)

Greater sciatic notch

B

plied paraspinal muscles take their origin from the iliac crest itself, as does the latissimus dorsi, which is supplied proximally by the long thoracic nerve. Thus, an incision into the iliac crest does not denervate muscles even if the incision is not exactly on the outer lip of the crest.

SUPERFICIAL SURGICAL DISSECTION

Dissect the subcutaneous tissues until you reach the iliac crest. In children, the iliac apophysis is white and quite visible; you may incise or split it in line with the iliac crest, using it as an avascular plane. In adults, the apophysis is ossified and fused to the crest; the incision lands you directly onto the crest itself.

Use the Cobb elevator to remove the apophysis or muscles from the iliac crest both medially and laterally, to bare the surface of the posterior portion of the crest.

DANGERS

Nerves

The **clunial nerves** cross the iliac crest. You can avoid them as long as you do not incise more than 8 cm anteriolateral to the posterior superior iliac spine. The nerves supply sensation to the skin over

the clunial (gluteal) area. They are composed of the posterior primary rami of L1, L2, and L3. Their loss does not cause problems for the patient.

DEEP SURGICAL DISSECTION

Completely strip the musculature off the posterior portion of the lateral surface of the ilium so that you can obtain a large enough graft. Take care to stay in a subperiosteal plane as you pass from the iliac crest to the outer cortex of the ilium. As you proceed 1.5 cm down the ilium in the area of the posterior superior spine, you will see and feel the elevated posterior gluteal line; pass subperiosteally up over the line and then down its other side. Do not err by letting the line direct you outward from bone into muscle. A Taylor retractor will help your exposure by holding the muscles laterally. Note that the posterior gluteal line separates the origins of the gluteus maximus (posterior) from the gluteus medius (anterior) (Fig. 6-110*A* and *B*).

DANGERS

Nerves

It is remotely possible that an osteotome will hit the **sciatic nerve,** which runs close to the distal end of the wound deep to the sciatic notch; however, if you draw an imaginary line from the posterior superior iliac spine perpendicular to the operating table and stay cephalad to it, you will completely avoid both notch and nerve. If you have to take a larger graft, palpate the sciatic notch itself before taking the graft (see Fig. 6-110B).

Vessels

The **superior gluteal vessel,** a branch of the internal iliac (hypogastric) artery, leaves the pelvis via the sciatic notch, staying against the bone and proximal to the piriformis muscle. If a graft is taken too close to the sciatic notch, the vessel may be cut and may retract into the pelvis. Nutrient vessels from the artery supply the iliac crest bone along the midportion of the anterior gluteal line, and the vessel may become an osseous bleeder as it enters bone via the nutrient foramen. To control bone bleeding, use bone wax on the raw cancellous surface of the pelvis after you have removed the graft.

Bone

Avoid the **sciatic notch.** Breaking through the thick portion of the bone that forms the notch disrupts the stability of the pelvis. Removal of bone from the false pelvis proximal to the notch does not cause loss of stability (see Fig. 6-110B).

HOW TO ENLARGE THE APPROACH

Local Measures

Place a sharp-tipped, right-angled Taylor retractor into the bone to retract the gluteal muscles away from the bone and increase the exposure. To further increase the exposure, lengthen the iliac crest incision and strip more of the gluteal muscles from the outer cortex so that you are not working through a "keyhole."

Extensile Measures

The incision is not extensile. It is specifically designed for removal of bone for graft material from the posterior outer cortex of the ilium. Inner cortex also may be taken.

ANTERIOR APPROACH TO THE ILIAC CREST FOR BONE GRAFT

Anterior iliac crest bone grafts are usually taken during anterior surgical procedures that include spinal fusion. The anterior iliac bone graft is most frequently used for anterior fusions of the cervical spine and lower lumbar spine, L5–S1. The bone grafts are usually taken from the posterior aspect of the iliac crest.

POSITION OF PATIENT

Place the patient supine on the operating table. Because the graft is usually taken in conjunction with other procedures, the iliac crest should be draped as a separate unit. Place a small sandbag under the gluteal (clunial) area of the side from which the graft is taken to elevate and internally rotate the crest, making it more accessible.

LANDMARKS AND INCISION

Landmarks

The subcutaneous *anterior superior iliac spine,* the most important landmark, is easily palpable. Continue palpating along the crest of the ilium until you come to the widest portion of the ilium, at the *iliac tubercle.* The iliac tubercle marks the anterior portion of the ilium, the area containing the largest amount of cortical cancellous bone for graft material.

Incision

Make an 8-cm incision parallel to the iliac crest and centered over the iliac tubercle (Fig. 6-111).

INTERNERVOUS PLANE

Muscles either take origin or insert onto the iliac crest but do not cross it. Therefore, the crest offers a truly internervous plane.

The tensor fasciae latae, the gluteus minimus, and the gluteus medius are the muscles most directly affected by grafts taken from the anterior portion of the crest, since they originate from the outer portion of the ilium and are supplied by the superior gluteal nerve. The abdominal muscles take their origin directly from the iliac crest and are segmentally supplied.

SUPERFICIAL SURGICAL DISSECTION

Retract the skin and identify the iliac crest. Incise the crest before releasing the muscle attachments.

In children, the crest may still be an avascular apophysis. If so, incise it and remove the muscles

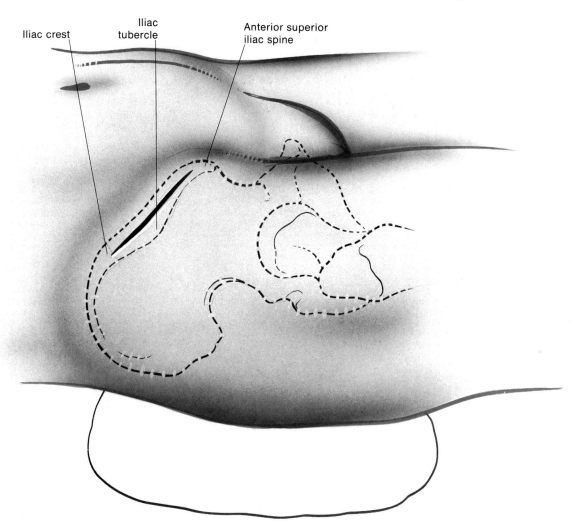

Iliac crest

Iliac
tubercle

Anterior superior
iliac spine

FIG. 6-111. Make an 8-cm incision parallel to the iliac crest and centered over the iliac tubercle.

from the crest in either direction with a Cobb elevator (Fig. 6-112).

Take care not to carry your incision from the apophysis or iliac crest onto the anterior superior iliac spine itself; if you do, you may detach the origin of the inguinal ligament and cause an inguinal hernia.

DEEP SURGICAL DISSECTION

After identifying the iliac crest and the iliac tubercle, remove the origins of the gluteus minimus and medius muscles subperiosteally from the outer cortex with Cobb elevators (Fig. 6-113). Note that the plane created is avascular. Bone may be taken in the form of dowel or block grafts. If you must, you can take graft from both cortices.

DANGERS

Both the crest of the ilium and the anterior superior iliac spine should be left intact to preserve

the normal appearance of the pelvis. If the anterior superior iliac spine is taken as graft, the inguinal ligament might retract, causing an inguinal hernia.

HOW TO ENLARGE THE APPROACH

Local Measures

Place a sharp-tipped Taylor retractor into the bone to retract the gluteal muscles from the outer cortex and to give a clearer view of the wound. You may have to lengthen the incision into the iliac crest and strip off additional amounts of gluteus medius muscle to get a better view of the outer cortex of the anterior portion of the ilium.

Extensile Measures

This incision is not extensile. It is specifically designed for removing bone from the anterior, outer, and inner cortices of the ilium.

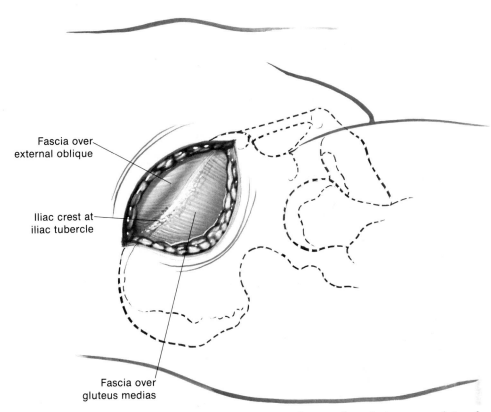

Fascia over
external oblique

Iliac crest at
iliac tubercle

Fascia over
gluteus medias

FIG. 6-112. Retract the skin, identify the iliac crest, and incise the soft tissues overlying the iliac crest down to bone.

FIG. 6-113. Remove the origins of the gluteus minimus and medius muscles subperiosteally from the outer cortex of the ilium.

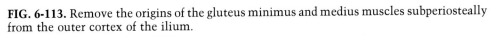

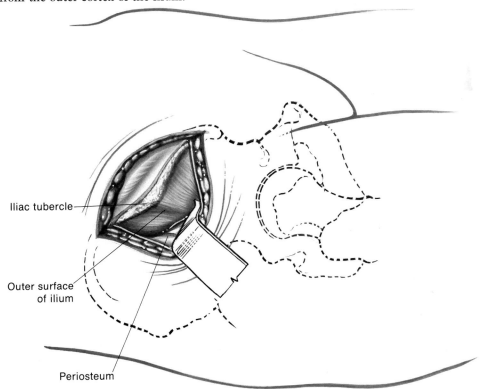

Iliac tubercle

Outer surface
of ilium

Periosteum

REFERENCES

1. MIXTER WJ, BARR JS: Rupture of the intervertebral disc and involvement of the spinal cord. N Engl J Med 211:210, 1934
2. SEIMON L: Low Back Pain: Clinical Diagnosis and Management. New York, Appleton-Century-Crofts, 1983
3. HIBBS RA: An operation for progressive spinal deformities. NY Med J 93:1013, 1911
4. HIBBS RA: A report of 59 cases of scoliosis treated by fusion operation. J Bone Joint Surg 6:3, 1924
5. ROTHMAN HR, SIMEONE FA: The Spine. Philadelphia, WB Saunders, 1975
6. HOLSCHER EC: Vascular complication of disc surgery. J Bone Joint Surg (Am) 30:968, 1948
7. SACKS S: Anterior interbody fusion of the lumbar spine: Indications and results in 200 cases. Clin Orthop 44:163, 1966
8. MICHELE AA, KRUEGER FJ: Surgical approach to the vertebral body. J Bone Joint Surg (Am) 31:873, 1949
9. PEARL FL: Muscle-splitting extra peritoneal lumbar ganglionectomy. Surg Gynecol Obstet 65:197, 1937
10. JOHNSON RM, SOUTHWICK WO: Surgical Approaches to the Cervical Spine, p. 133–1–10 to 1–32.
11. ROGERS WA: Treatment of fracture dislocation of the cervical spine. J Bone Joint Surg 24:245, 1942
12. HOLDSWORTH FW: Fractures, dislocations and fracture dislocations of the spine. J Bone Joint Surg (Br) 45:6, 1963
13. WILLARD DP, NICHOLSON JT: Dislocations of the first cervical vertebra. Ann Surg 113:464, 1941
14. CLOWARD RB: Personal communication, 1969
15. ROBINSON, RA, SMITH GW: Anterolateral cervical disc removal and interbody fusion for cervical disc syndrome. Bull Johns Hopkins Hosp 96:223, 1955
16. HOPPENFELD S: Physical Examination of the Spine & Extremities, p 107. New York, Appleton-Century-Crofts, 1976
17. CAPENER N: The evolution of lateral rhachotomy. J Bone Joint Surg (Br) 36:173, 1954
18. WILKINSON MC: Curettage of tuberculous vertebral disease in treatment of spinal caries. Proc R Soc Med 43:114, 1950
19. BURCH BH, MILLER AC: Atlas of Pulmonary Resections, pp 8–11. Springfield, IL, Charles C Thomas, 1965
20. COOK WA: Trans-thoracic vertebral surgery. Ann Thorac Surg 12:54, 1971
21. HODGSON AR, STOCK FE, FANG HSY ET AL: Anterior spinal fusion: The operative approach and pathological findings in 412 patients with Pott's disease of the spine. Br J Surg 48:172, 1980
22. HOPPENFELD S: A Manual of Concept and Treatment, pp 96–99. Philadelphia, JB Lippincott, 1967
23. WINTER RB: Congenital Deformities of the Spine. New York, Grune & Stratton, 1983
24. MOE J, WINTER RB, BRADFORD LONSTEIN J: Scoliosis and Spinal Deformities. Philadelphia, WB Saunders, 1978
25. KEIM H: The Adolescent Spine, p 159. New York, Grune & Stratton, 1976
26. HARRINGTON PR: Treatment of scoliosis: Correction and internal fixation by spine instrumentation. J Bone Joint Surg (Am) 44:591, 1962

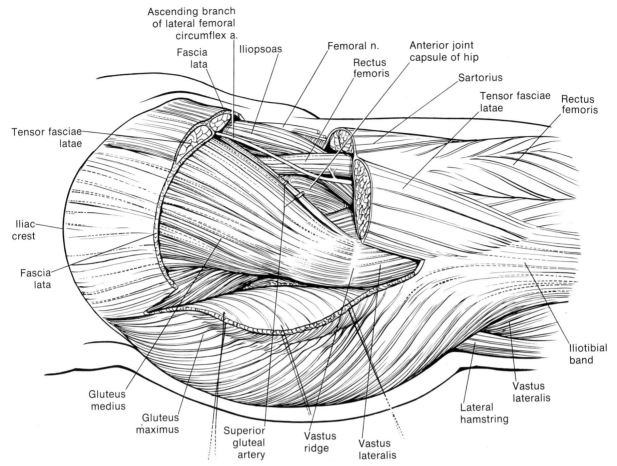

Ascending branch
of lateral femoral
circumflex a.

Fascia
lata

Iliopsoas

Femoral n.

Rectus
femoris

Anterior joint
capsule of hip

Sartorius

Tensor fasciae
latae

Rectus
femoris

Tensor fasciae
latae

Iliac
crest

Fascia
lata

Iliotibial
band

Gluteus
medius

Gluteus
maximus

Superior
gluteal
artery

Vastus
ridge

Vastus
lateralis

Lateral
hamstring

Vastus
lateralis

FIG. 7-34. Resecting the sartorius, tensor fasciae latae, and fascia lata and reflecting the anterior portion of the gluteus maximus posteriorly reveal the gluteus medius and more anterior structures of the hip region. The fascia lata splits to envelop the tensor fasciae latae, but it only covers the gluteus medius muscle.

Gluteus Medius. *Origin.* Outer aspect of ilium between anterior and posterior gluteal lines and its overlying fascia. *Insertion.* Lateral surface of greater trochanter. *Action.* Abductor and medial rotator of hip. *Nerve supply.* Superior gluteal nerve.

The origins of the external oblique and internal oblique are not detached during the anterior approach; the tensor fasciae latae is.

The *greater trochanter* is the traction apophysis of the proximal femur and the site of the insertion of the gluteus medius and minimus muscles. (See Posterior Approach.)

The *vastus lateralis ridge* results partly from the pull of the aponeurosis of the vastus lateralis during growth and partly from the fusion of the trochanter apophyses of the shaft of the femur (Fig. 7-36; see Fig. 7-34).

Incisions

Both anterior and anterolateral incisions largely ignore the lines of cleavage in the skin, but the scars are seldom broad and are nearly always hidden by clothing.

SUPERFICIAL SURGICAL DISSECTION AND ITS DANGERS

Both approaches use planes that involve the *tensor fasciae latae.* The anterior approach passes in front of it; the anterolateral approach passes behind it (Fig. 7-37).

Anterior Approach

The tensor fasciae latae and the sartorius run side by side from an almost continuous line of origin along the anterior end of the iliac crest. The two muscles diverge a short distance below the anterior superior iliac spine so that the rectus femoris can emerge from between them (see Fig. 7-14).

The *tensor fasciae latae* itself is triangular. In cross section, it is unusually slim at its origin and thick just before it inserts into the iliotibial tract.

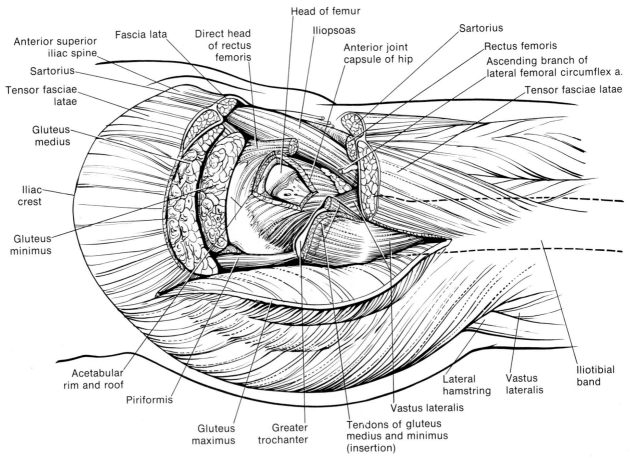

FIG. 7-35. The gluteus medius, gluteus minimus, and rectus femoris have been resected to reveal the muscular layers down to the hip joint capsule. Resection of the joint capsule exposes the acetabulum and the femoral head and neck.

FIG. 7-36. Osteology of the lateral aspect of the hip and pelvis.

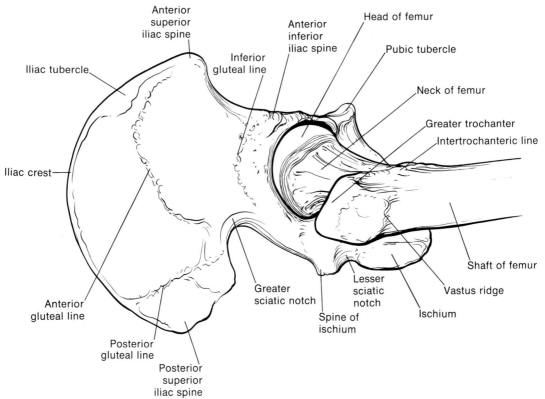

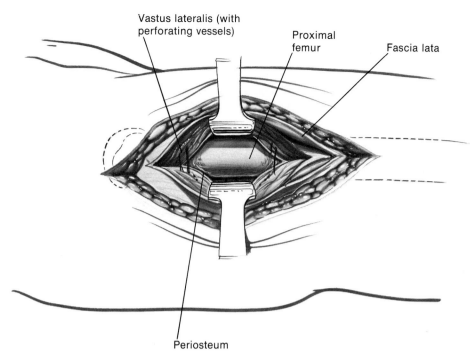

FIG. 8-5. Split the fibers of the vastus lateralis. To develop a subperiosteal plane, squeeze two Homan retractors down to the femoral shaft and separate them to split the vastus lateralis further.

FIG. 8-6. The incision may be extended distally to expose the entire shaft of the femur.

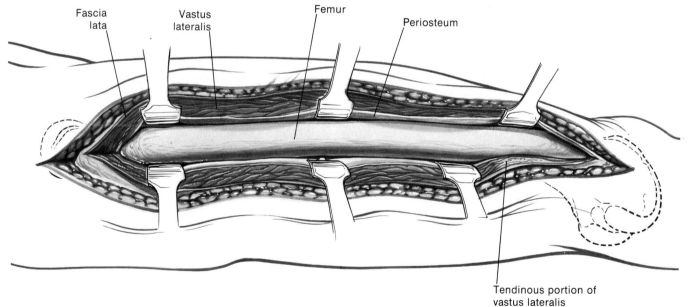

Continue splitting by blunt dissections. As you do so, you will expose several vessels that cross the field. Coagulate them, if possible, before they are avulsed by the blunt dissection.

Incise the periosteum on the lateral aspect of the femur; continue the dissection subperiosteally around the bone to reveal the femoral shaft. (This is seldom possible in elderly patients, in whom the periosteum is exceptionally thin, but it is very easy in children.)

DANGERS

Vessels

Numerous **perforating branches of the profunda femoris artery** traverse the vastus lateralis (see Fig. 8-35). They are damaged during the approach and should be ligated or coagulated. You can identify them more easily if you split the muscle gently with a blunt instrument rather than cut straight through it with a knife.

361

HOW TO ENLARGE THE APPROACH

Extensile Measures

The approach is most useful for exposing the proximal third of the bone for internal fixation of a hip fracture. However, it can be extended to the knee joint to allow full exposure of the lateral aspect of the femoral shaft for reduction and fixation of all types of femoral fractures (Fig. 8-6; see Figs. 8-34, and 8-35).

POSTEROLATERAL APPROACH

The posterolateral[1] approach can expose the entire length of the femur. Because it follows the lateral intermuscular septum, it does not interfere with the quadriceps muscle. While other lateral approaches involve splitting the vastus lateralis or the vastus intermedius, the functional results of the posterolateral approach do not differ significantly from them, probably because the vastus lateralis originates partly from the lateral intermuscular septum. As a result, surgery still involves detaching a part of the muscle's origin and does not use a true intermuscular plane.

The uses of the posterolateral approach include the following:

1. Open reduction and plating of femoral fractures, especially supracondylar fractures
2. Open intramedullary rodding of femoral shaft fractures
3. Treatment of nonunion of femoral fractures
4. Femoral osteotomy (rarely performed in the region of the femoral shaft)
5. Treatment of chronic or acute osteomyelitis
6. Biopsy and treatment of bone tumors

POSITION OF PATIENT

Place the patient supine on the operating table with a sandbag beneath the buttock on the affected side to elevate the buttock and to internally rotate the leg, bringing the posterolateral surface of the thigh clear of the table (Fig. 8-7).

LANDMARKS AND INCISION

Landmarks

Palpate the *lateral femoral epicondyle* on the lateral surface of the knee joint. The epicondyle is actually a flare of the condyle. As you move superiorly, note that you cannot palpate the femur above the epicondyle.

Incision

Make a longitudinal incision on the posterolateral aspect of the thigh. Base the distal part of the incision on the lateral femoral epicondyle and continue proximally along the posterior part of the femoral shaft. The exact length of the incision depends on the surgery to be performed (Fig. 8-9).

INTERNERVOUS PLANE

The approach exploits the plane between the *vastus lateralis* (femoral nerve) and the *lateral intermuscular septum*, which covers the *hamstring muscles* (sciatic nerve) (Fig. 8-8).

SUPERFICIAL SURGICAL DISSECTION

Incise the deep fascia of the thigh in line with its fibers and the skin incision (Fig. 8-10).

DEEP SURGICAL DISSECTION

Identify the vastus lateralis under the fascia lata (Fig. 8-11). Follow the muscle posteriorly to the lateral intermuscular septum. Now reflect the muscle anteriorly, dissecting between muscle and septum. Numerous branches of the perforating arteries cross this septum to supply the muscle; they must be ligated or coagulated (Fig. 8-12).

Continue the dissection, following the plane between the lateral intermuscular septum and the vastus lateralis, detaching those parts of the vastus lateralis that arise from the septum until you reach the femur at the linea aspera (Fig. 8-13). Incise the periosteum longitudinally at this point and strip off the muscles covering the femur by subperiosteal dissection. Detaching muscles from the linea aspera itself usually has to be done by sharp dissection (Fig. 8-14).

DANGERS

Vessels

The **perforating arteries** (branches of the profunda femoris artery) pierce the lateral intermuscular septum to supply the vastus lateralis muscle. They must be ligated or coagulated one by one as the dissection progresses. If they are torn flush with the lateral intermuscular septum, they may begin to bleed out of control as they retract behind the lateral intermuscular septum (see Fig. 8-35). *(Text continues on p. 366)*

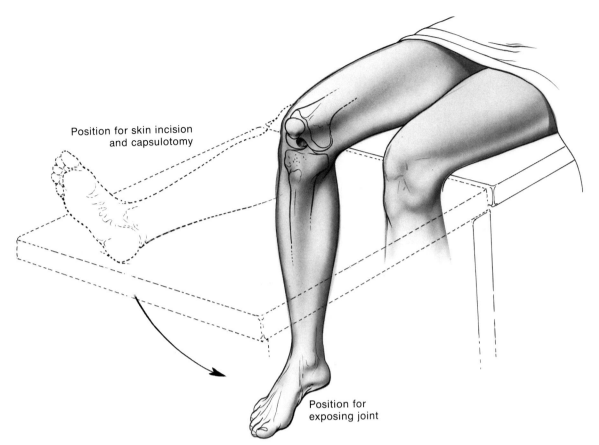

Position for skin incision
and capsulotomy

Position for
exposing joint

FIG. 9-1. Position of the patient for the medial parapatellar approach. Begin with the straight leg position; then flex the knee for the deeper dissection.

runs from the inferior border of the patella and is palpable to its insertion into the tibial tubercle.

Incisions

Begin the incision on the medial side of the quadriceps tendon and 3 cm to 5 cm above the superior pole of the patella. Run it distally to the superior medial corner and around the medial border of the patella. Then curve the incision anteriorly, running toward and just medial to the patellar ligament. The incision is usually 10 cm to 12 cm long but can be extended if necessary (Fig. 9-2).

Alternatively, for joint replacement surgery, make a longitudinal, straight, midline incision extending from a point 5 cm above the patella to below the level of the tibial tubercle (see Fig. 9-2).

A medial parapatellar capsular incision completes the deep dissection for both skin incisions (Fig. 9-3).

INTERNERVOUS PLANE

There is no internervous plane in this approach, even when the incision is extended superiorly into the intermuscular plane between the vastus medialis and the rectus femoris. Both of these muscles are supplied by the femoral nerve well proximal to this dissection, leaving the plane safe for knee surgery.

SUPERFICIAL SURGICAL DISSECTION

Continue cutting through the joint capsule and along the patellar ligament and quadriceps tendon in line with the original skin incision. Take care to leave a cuff of capsular tissue medial to the patella and lateral to the quadriceps to facilitate closure. Incise the synovium in the same line as the capsular incision, from the suprapatellar pouch to just below the joint line. Retract the fat pad or incise it with cautery, as dictated by your exposure requirements. As you approach the joint line, take care not to damage the anterior insertion of the medial meniscus (Fig. 9-4).

When total joint replacement is contemplated, a straight midline incision is thought to be associated with fewer postoperative complications. Develop a medial skin flap just enough to leave room for a medial parapatellar capsular incision.

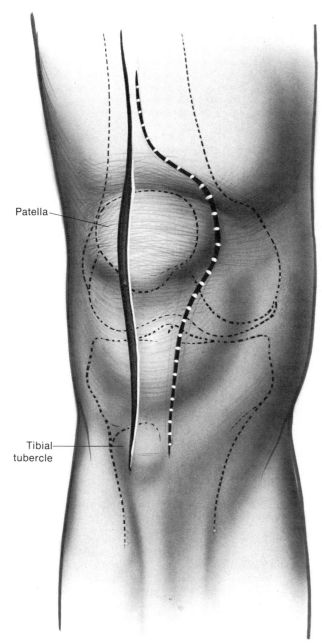

FIG. 9-2. Two incisions are possible: a parapatellar skin incision with proximal and distal extensions, or a longitudinal, straight, midline incision.

Then continue the capsular incision as described (see Figs. 9-2 and 9-3).

DEEP SURGICAL DISSECTION

Dislocate the patella laterally and rotate it 180°, then flex the knee to 90° (Fig. 9-5; see Fig. 9-1). Try to avoid avulsing the patellar ligament from its insertion on the tibia as you dislocate the patella, since reattaching the tendon to the bone is difficult. If the patella does not dislocate easily, you can give it added mobility in two ways:

1. Extend the skin incision superiorly over the interval between the rectus femoris and the vastus medialis. Continue the dissection deeper, splitting the quadriceps tendon farther just lateral to its medial border (see Fig. 9-5).
2. Carefully reflect the proximal half of the patellar ligament insertion by subperiosteal dissection (Fig. 9-6A).

If you are faced with one of those rare cases in which the patella still does not dislocate, carefully remove the patellar ligament attachment with an underlying block of bone. The bone makes subsequent reattachment easier (Fig. 9-6B).

When the patella is dislocated and the knee is fully flexed, this incision gives the widest possible exposure of the entire knee joint.

DANGERS

Nerves

The **infrapatellar branch of the saphenous nerve** is often cut during this approach. Transection is more likely to occur with parapatellar than with midline skin incisions. The major danger in cutting the nerve is the development of a postoperative neuroma. Because the area of anesthesia produced is usually not troublesome, do not repair the nerve if you cut it. Instead, resect it and bury its end in fat to decrease the chances that a painful neuroma will form (see Fig. 9-24 and Fig. 9-27).

Muscles and Ligaments

If the patellar ligament becomes avulsed from its insertion on the tibia, it is difficult to reattach.

HOW TO ENLARGE THE APPROACH

Local Measures

SUPERIOR EXTENSION. Extend the approach proximally between the rectus femoris and the vastus medialis. Then split the underlying vastus intermedius to expose the distal two thirds of the femur. Stay in the distal third of the thigh; more proximally, you may involve the branches of the femoral nerve and cause partial denervation (see pp. 370–373).

INFERIOR EXTENSION. Mobilize the upper part of the attachment of the patellar ligament to the tibia or remove the patellar ligament with a underlying block of bone. This extension may be useful in dealing with complex intra-articular fractures of the knee joint. (See Lateral Approach to the Distal Femur for combined use in repair of the cruciate ligament.)

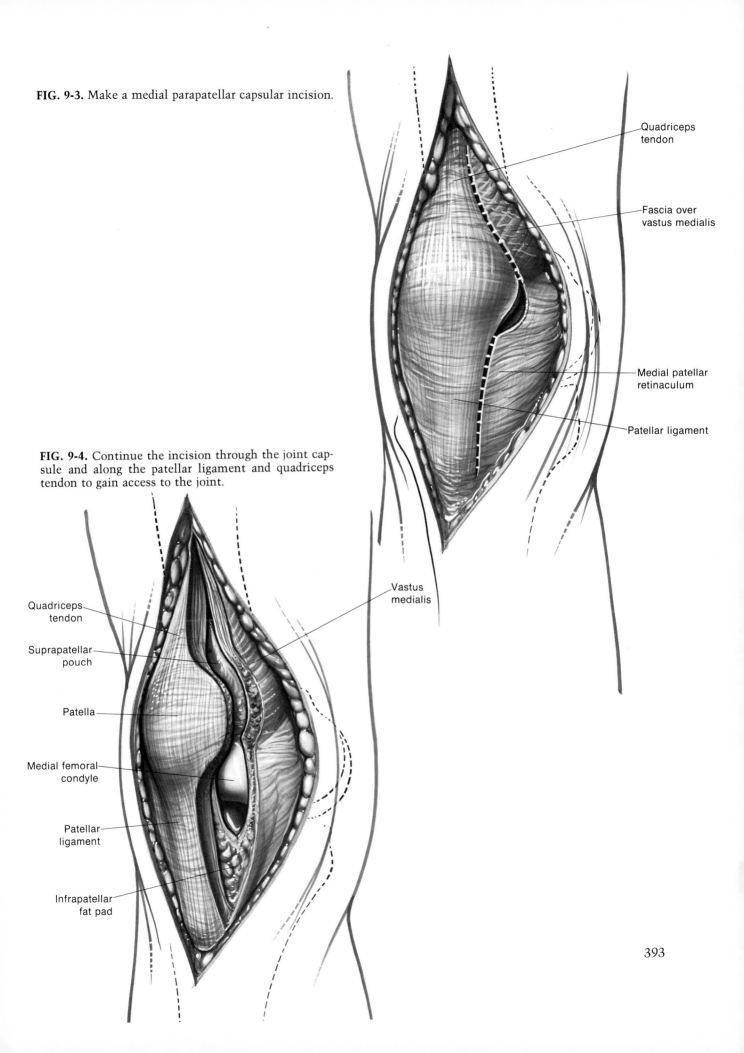

FIG. 9-3. Make a medial parapatellar capsular incision.

Quadriceps
tendon

Fascia over
vastus medialis

Medial patellar
retinaculum

Patellar ligament

FIG. 9-4. Continue the incision through the joint capsule and along the patellar ligament and quadriceps tendon to gain access to the joint.

Vastus
medialis

Quadriceps
tendon

Suprapatellar
pouch

Patella

Medial femoral
condyle

Patellar
ligament

Infrapatellar
fat pad

393

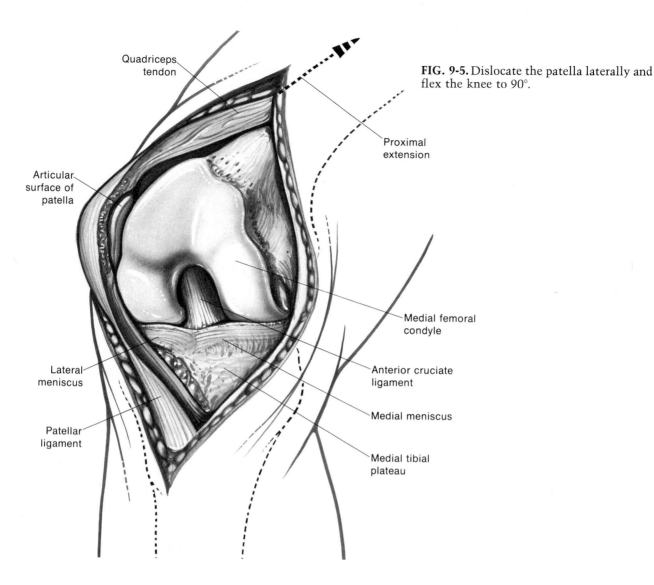

FIG. 9-5. Dislocate the patella laterally and flex the knee to 90°.

Quadriceps tendon

Proximal extension

Articular surface of patella

Medial femoral condyle

Anterior cruciate ligament

Lateral meniscus

Medial meniscus

Patellar ligament

Medial tibial plateau

FIG. 9-6. Measures to facilitate patellar dislocation. **(A)** detach the proximal half of the patellar ligament insertion. **(B)** Detach the patellar ligament attachment with an underlying block of bone.

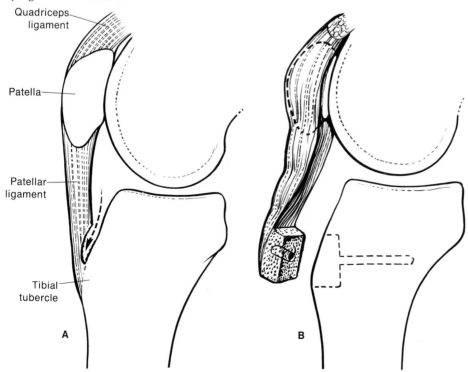

Quadriceps ligament

Patella

Patellar ligament

Tibial tubercle

A

B

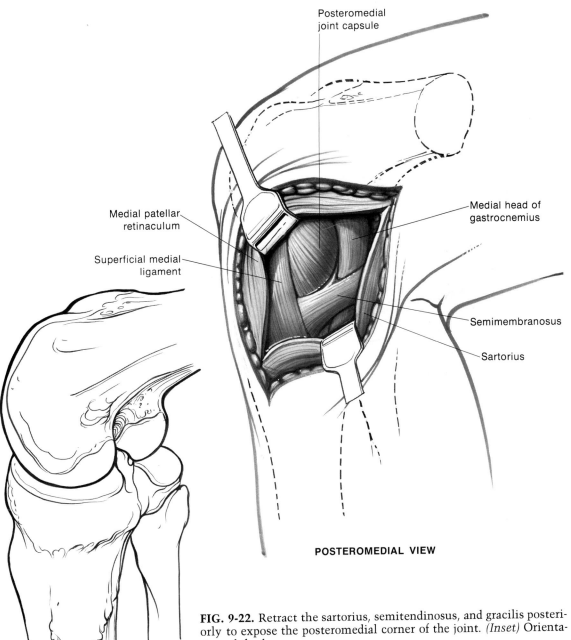

Posteromedial
joint capsule

Medial patellar
retinaculum

Superficial medial
ligament

Medial head of
gastrocnemius

Semimembranosus

Sartorius

POSTEROMEDIAL VIEW

FIG. 9-22. Retract the sartorius, semitendinosus, and gracilis posteriorly to expose the posteromedial corner of the joint. *(Inset)* Orientation of the knee.

receives its nerve supply well proximal to the approach and the gastrocnemius well distal.

Finally, separate the medial head of the gastrocnemius from the posterior capsule of the knee joint almost to the midline by blunt dissection (Fig. 9-23). Full exposure allows you to inspect the posteromedial corner of the capsule for damage. A second arthrotomy posterior to the superficial medial ligament (tibial collateral ligament) permits inspection or treatment of posterior intra-articular or periarticular pathology (see Fig.

9-23). Repair of the posteromedial corner of the joint is also possible.

DANGERS

Nerves

The cut end of the **infrapatellar branch of the saphenous nerve** should be buried in fat to prevent the formation of a postoperative neuroma.

The saphenous nerve emerges from between the

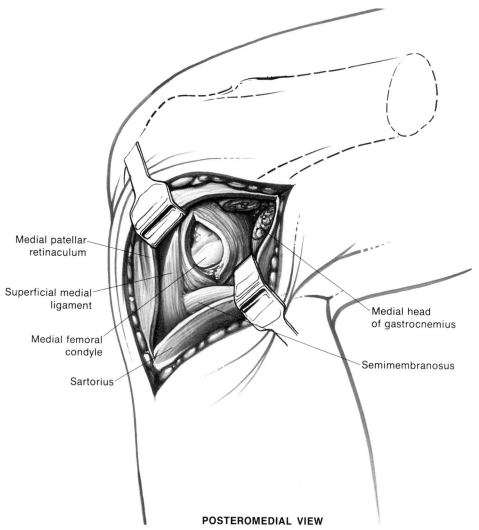

Medial patellar retinaculum

Superficial medial ligament

Medial femoral condyle

Sartorius

Medial head of gastrocnemius

Semimembranosus

POSTEROMEDIAL VIEW

FIG. 9-23. Expose the posteromedial corner of the knee joint by first separating the gastrocnemius and the posterior capsule of the joint and then performing a capsulotomy posterior to the tibial collateral ligament.

gracilis and the sartorius and runs with the long saphenous vein. It provides sensation for some of the non-weight-bearing portions of the foot and should be preserved (see Figs. 9-24 and 9-27).

Vessels

The **saphenous vein** appears in the posterior corner of the superficial dissection. Because it may be required for future vascular procedures, it should be preserved (see Fig. 9-27).

The **medial inferior genicular artery** curves around the upper end of the tibia. It may be damaged when the medial belly of the gastrocnemius is lifted off the posterior capsule: the damage may go unnoticed until the wound is closed and the tourniquet is released (see Figs. 9-30 and 9-31).

The **popliteal artery** lies against the posterior joint capsule in the midline and is adjacent to the

medial head of the gastrocnemius. Take care to avoid injuring the vessel when you separate the gastrocnemius from the joint capsule (see Figs. 9-50 and 9-53).

SPECIAL PROBLEMS

Hematomas under the skin flap that develop postoperatively can cause skin necrosis. Therefore, the large skin flaps created in this approach should be well drained.

HOW TO ENLARGE THE APPROACH

The incision is already extensive, giving exposure to all the medial structures of the knee, and cannot be usefully extended in either direction. (For repair of the anterior cruciate ligament, see Lateral Approach to the Distal Femur.)

APPLIED SURGICAL ANATOMY OF THE MEDIAL SIDE OF THE KNEE

OVERVIEW

As Warren and Marshall pointed out, the ligaments on the medial side of the knee are merely "condensations within tissue planes."[15] They blend with each other at various points, making definition of each layer difficult, even more so in cases of trauma, when bleeding and edema can further complicate the problem. For this reason, it is important to have a concept of the normal anatomy and the supporting structures on the medial side of the knee.

The anatomy of the medial side is readily understood when it is described in three separate layers.[15] Approaches to the knee enter the joint by sequentially incising these layers, from outside to inside.

Outer Layer

The outer layer consists of the proximal continuation of the deep fascia of the thigh. It encloses the sartorius muscle, whose fibers blend with the fascial layer before they insert into the tibia.

Anteriorly, the outer layer blends with fibrous tissue derived from the vastus medialis to form the medial patellar retinaculum. Posteriorly, the layer is continuous with the deep fascia, which covers the gastrocnemius and the roof of the popliteal fossa (Figs. 9-24 and 9-27).

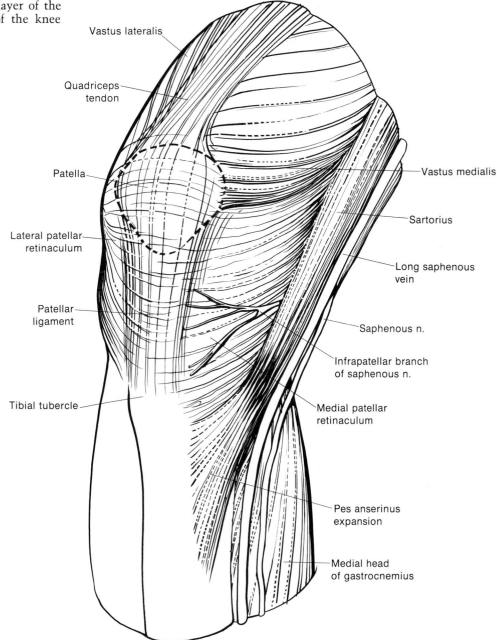

FIG. 9-24. The outer layer of the anteromedial aspect of the knee joint.

Vastus lateralis

Quadriceps tendon

Patella

Lateral patellar retinaculum

Patellar ligament

Tibial tubercle

Vastus medialis

Sartorius

Long saphenous vein

Saphenous n.

Infrapatellar branch of saphenous n.

Medial patellar retinaculum

Pes anserinus expansion

Medial head of gastrocnemius

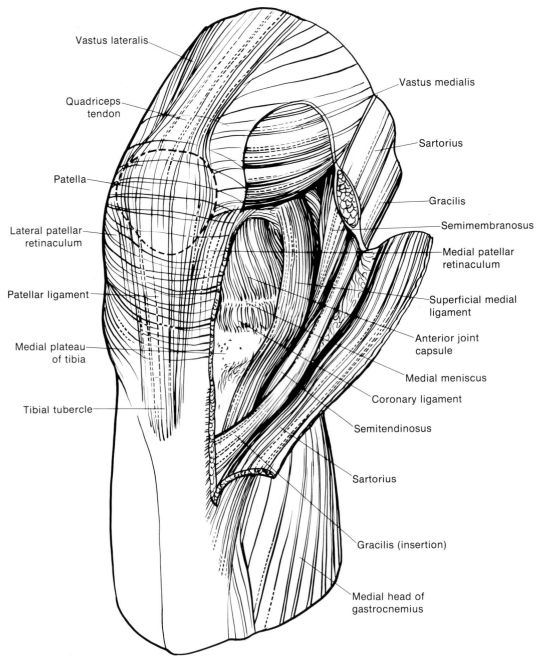

Vastus lateralis

Quadriceps tendon

Patella

Lateral patellar retinaculum

Patellar ligament

Medial plateau of tibia

Tibial tubercle

Vastus medialis

Sartorius

Gracilis

Semimembranosus

Medial patellar retinaculum

Superficial medial ligament

Anterior joint capsule

Medial meniscus

Coronary ligament

Semitendinosus

Sartorius

Gracilis (insertion)

Medial head of gastrocnemius

FIG. 9-25. The sartorius and the medial patellar retinaculum (outer layer) have been resected to reveal the superficial medial ligament of the middle layer. The true joint capsule (deep layer) is also exposed.

Middle Layer

The middle layer consists of the superficial medial ligament (tibial or medial collateral ligament), which is attached superiorly just below the adductor tubercle of the femur. The ligament, which is quadrangular, fans out as it travels down to insert into the subcutaneous border of the tibia

some 6 cm to 7 cm below the knee joint. It lies behind the axis of rotation of the knee (Figs. 9-25 and 9-26).

Above the superficial medial ligament, fibrous tissue from the middle layer passes to the medial side of the patella, forming the medial patellofemoral ligament (see Fig. 9-26).

FIG. 9-32. Osteology of the posteromedial aspect of the knee joint.

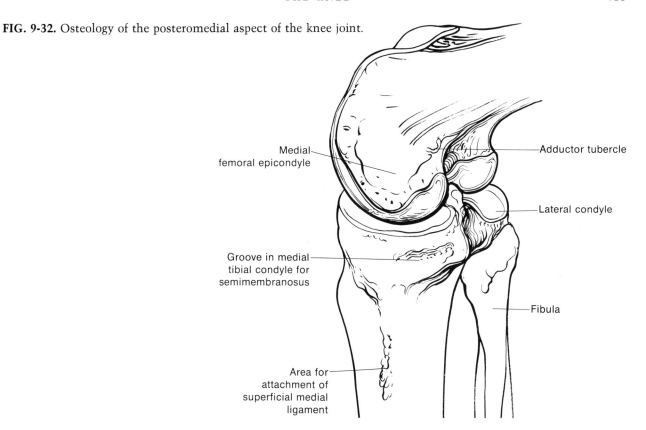

SPECIAL ANATOMICAL POINTS

Three muscles, the sartorius, the semitendinosus, and the gracilis, insert into the upper part of the subcutaneous surface of the tibia. Each muscle has a different nerve supply: The sartorius is innervated by the femoral nerve, the semitendinosus by the sciatic nerve, and the gracilis by the obturator nerve. In addition, each muscle crosses both the hip and the knee

The actions of the three muscles are duplicated by other, more powerful, muscles. At their pelvic origins, the three attach to three points on the bony pelvis that are as widely separated as the pelvis allows: the anterior superior iliac spine (sartorius), the ischial tuberosity (semitendinosus), and the inferior pubic ramus (gracilis). With these origins and insertions, the muscles are ideally arranged to stabilize the pelvis on the leg.

The sartorius, semitendinosus, and gracilis insert into the subcutaneous surface of the tibia at a point called the *pes anserinus* (goose foot). Acting together, they not only flex the knee but also internally rotate the tibia.

APPROACH FOR LATERAL MENISCECTOMY

A lateral meniscectomy can be performed through several types of incisions. Longitudinal and oblique incisions give better access to other structures within the joint, while a transverse incision gives limited access to the knee but excellent exposure of the meniscus itself. All incisions enter the lateral compartment of the knee anterior to the superficial lateral ligament.

The approach is used for the following:

1. Lateral meniscectomy, total and partial[16]
2. Removal of loose bodies
3. Removal of foreign bodies
4. Treatment of osteochondritis of the lateral femoral condyle

POSITION OF PATIENT

Table Bent Position

The table bent position is identical to that used for medial meniscectomy (see p. 391). Two points are critical:

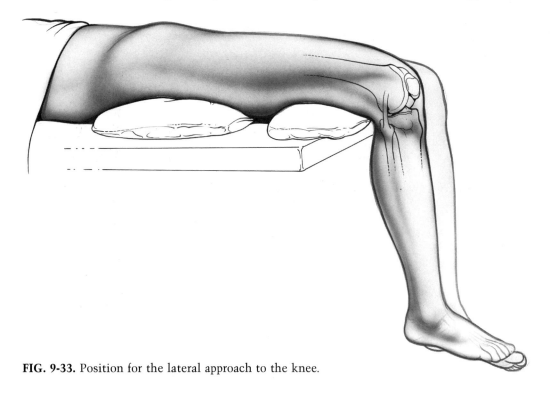

FIG. 9-33. Position for the lateral approach to the knee.

FIG. 9-34. With the patient supine on the operating table, drop the end of the table so the knee can flex. The cross-leg position allows a direct approach to the lateral aspect of the knee.

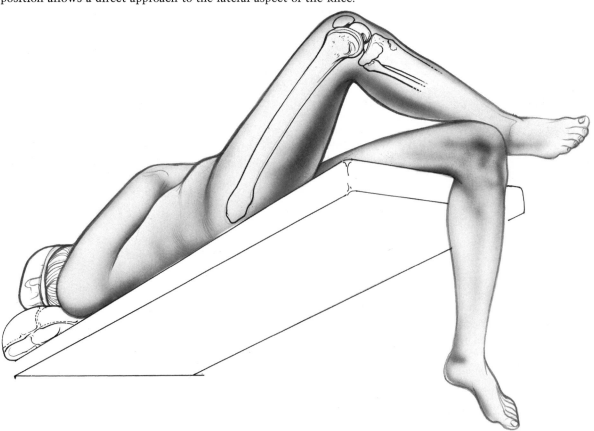

1. The sandbag must be placed under the thigh, not under the knee, to keep the popliteal artery and the posterior capsule from being compressed against the back of the femur and tibia.
2. The knee should be free to flex more than 90° to allow the best possible access to the back of the joint (Fig. 9-33).

Cross-Leg Position

Place the patient supine on the operating table. Drop the end of the table so the knees can flex. Then place the calf of the affected side over the opposite thigh to flex the affected knee and to abduct and externally rotate the hip. Now, place the table in 45° of Trendelenburg to bring the lateral side of the knee up to eye level. Finally, flex the head of the table up so that the patient does not slide backward (Fig. 9-34).

For both positions, exsanguinate the limb either by elevating it for 2 minutes or by applying a soft rubber bandage. Next, inflate a tourniquet.

LANDMARKS AND INCISION

Landmarks

The *lateral femoral condyle* is palpable along its smooth surface as far as the joint line.

The *head of the fibula* is situated at about the same level as the tibial tubercle. From the lateral femoral epicondyle, move your thumb inferiorly and posteriorly across the joint line to find it.

Palpate the *lateral border of the patella.*

To find the *lateral joint line,* flex and extend the knee; palpate the hinge area with your thumb to feel the movement of the femur and the tibia.

To palpate the *superficial lateral ligament (fibular collateral ligament,* lateral collateral ligament), cross the patient's leg so that his ankle rests on the opposite knee. When the knee is flexed to 90° and the hip is abducted and externally rotated, the iliotibial tract relaxes and makes the superficial lateral ligament easier to isolate. The ligament stands away from the joint itself, stretching from the fibular head to the lateral femoral condyle.

Incision

Of all the skin incisions around the knee, the oblique incision gives the most leeway, both for meniscectomies and for other intra-articular procedures, should they prove necessary. To make the incision, start at the inferolateral corner of the patella and continue downward and backward for about 5 cm. The cut should remain considerably anterior to the superficial lateral ligament, which lies under a line drawn vertically up from the head

of the fibula to the lateral femoral condyle (Fig. 9-35A).

INTERNERVOUS PLANE

There is no internervous plane in this approach, which consists mainly of incisions of the lateral patellar retinaculum and the joint capsule. No major nerves are in or near the area.

SUPERFICIAL SURGICAL DISSECTION

Open the anterolateral aspect of the knee capsule in line with the incision (Fig. 9-35B).

DEEP SURGICAL DISSECTION

Incise the synovium and extrasynovial fat of the knee joint in line with the incision to open the anterolateral portion of the joint. To avoid damaging the underlying meniscus, begin the incision well above the joint line and cut down carefully (Figs. 9-35C and 9-36).

DANGERS

Vessels

The **lateral inferior genicular artery** runs around the upper part of the tibia. The artery lies next to the peripheral attachment of the lateral meniscus; it may be damaged if the meniscus is detached along a portion of the capsule during meniscectomy, leading to massive postoperative hemarthrosis. It is not in danger during the approach (see Fig. 9-42).

Muscles and Ligaments

The **superficial lateral ligament** (fibular collateral ligament) limits posterior extension at the incision. If it is cut and not repaired, it may affect lateral stability. Its position may be estimated by a line drawn from the head of the fibula to the lateral femoral condyle (see Fig. 9-42).

SPECIAL PROBLEMS

The lateral meniscus may be damaged if the synovium is incised too close to the joint line.

HOW TO ENLARGE THE APPROACH

This particular approach restricts the view of the inside of the joint because of the relative immobility of the structures that are incised and the difficulty in retracting them. There are three ways to improve the exposure without extending the incision:

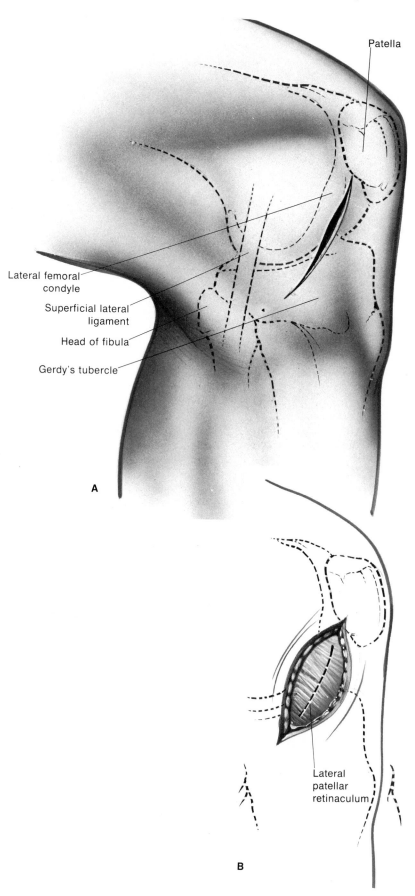

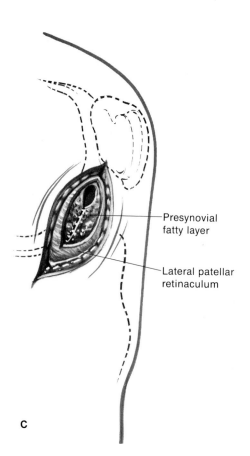

FIG. 9-35

(A) Incision for the lateral approach to the knee. The incision should remain considerably anterior to the superficial lateral (fibular collateral) ligament.

(B) Incise the knee joint capsule in line with the skin incision.

(C) Incise the synovium and extrasynovial fat pad to enter the joint. Avoid damaging the underlying meniscus.

FIG. 9-36. Expose the meniscus. Place retractors to allow maximum exposure of the joint.

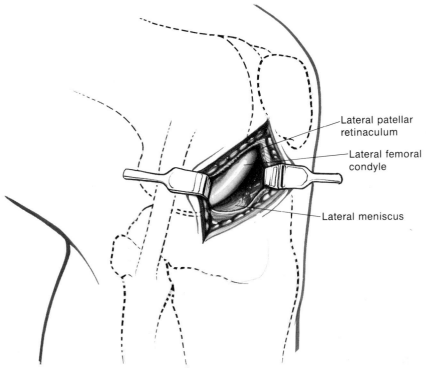

Lateral patellar retinaculum

Lateral femoral condyle

Lateral meniscus

1. *Retraction.* Retractors should be readjusted frequently to allow the best possible view.
2. *Position of joint.* A varus stress opens up the lateral side of the joint, one advantage of the cross-leg position, which automatically puts a varus stress on the knee. Flexion of the knee allows better access to the back of the lateral side of the joint.
3. *Lights.* The direction of the light should be adjusted frequently so that it shines into the depths of the wound. A headlamp can be used to advantage for lateral meniscectomies.

Extensile Measures

POSTERIOR EXTENSION.   The incision cannot be extended posteriorly because of the presence of the superficial lateral ligament.

SUPERIOR EXTENSION. To extend the incision superiorly, incise the skin and lateral patellar retinaculum along the lateral border of the patella, increasing access to the back of the patella. To widen the exposure still further, extend the incision superiorly and open the plane between the vastus lateralis and the rectus femoris. Broadening the approach to an anterolateral approach to the femur offers the theoretical possibility of extending the exposure as far as the anterior superior iliac spine (see pp. 366–369).

LATERAL APPROACH TO THE KNEE AND ITS SUPPORTING STRUCTURES

The lateral approach gives access to all the supporting structures on the lateral side of the knee. It may be extended for intra-articular exploration of the knee's anterior and posterior structures as well.

Normally, only part of the exposure is needed for any single piece of surgery. Its major use is in assessment of ligamentous damage, pathology that is more common on the medial side, since valgus stress is more common than varus stress.

POSITION OF PATIENT

Place the patient supine on the operating table with a sandbag under the buttock of the affected side. This position rotates the leg medially to better expose the lateral aspect of the knee. Flex the knee to 90°. Exsanguinate the limb either by elevating it for 3 to 5 minutes or by applying a soft rubber bandage; then inflate a tourniquet (see Fig. 9-33).

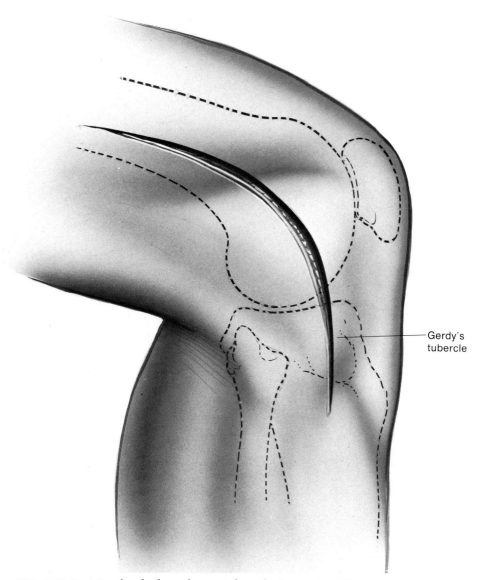

FIG. 9-37. Incision for the lateral approach to the knee joint. The incision should be made with the knee flexed.

LANDMARKS AND INCISION

Landmarks

Locate the *lateral border of the patella* and the *lateral joint line.*

Gerdy's tubercle (lateral tubercle of the tibia), a smooth, circular facet on the anterior surface of the lateral condyle of the tibia, marks the inferior attachment of the iliotibial band. Palpate it just lateral to the patellar ligament.

Incision

A long, curved incision is needed for adequate exposure of all the knee's lateral structures. Begin the incision at the level of the middle of the patella and 3 cm lateral to it. With the knee still flexed, extend the cut downward, over Gerdy's tubercle on the tibia and 4 cm to 5 cm distal to the joint line. Complete the incision by curving its upper end to follow the line of the femur (Fig. 9-37).

INTERNERVOUS PLANE

The dissection exploits the plane between the *iliotibial band* and the *biceps femoris*. The iliotibial band is the fascial aponeurosis of two muscles, the gluteus maximus and the tensor fasciae latae, both of which are supplied by the superior gluteal nerve. The biceps femoris is supplied by the sciatic nerve. Although the iliotibial band itself has no nerve supply, the plane between it and the biceps femoris can be considered an internervous one because of the band's muscular origin (Fig. 9-38).

SUPERFICIAL SURGICAL DISSECTION

Mobilize the skin flaps widely. Underneath are two major structures: the iliotibial band, sweeping down to attach to the anterolateral border of the tibia and Gerdy's tubercle, and the biceps femoris, passing downward and forward to attach to the head of the fibula. Both of these structures may be avulsed from their insertions in severe varus stress to the knee.

Incise the fascia in the interval between the iliotibial band and the biceps femoris, avoiding the common peroneal nerve on the biceps tendon's posterior border (Fig. 9-39). Retract the iliotibial band anteriorly and the biceps femoris (with the peroneal nerve) posteriorly, uncovering the superficial lateral (fibular collateral) ligament as it runs from the lateral epicondyle of the femur to the head of the fibula. The posterolateral corner of the knee capsule is also visible (Fig. 9-40).

DEEP SURGICAL DISSECTION

Enter the joint either in front of or behind the superficial lateral ligament (see Fig. 9-40).

Anterior Arthrotomy

To inspect the entire lateral meniscus, incise the capsule in front of the ligament. Make a separate fascial incision to create a lateral parapatellar approach. To avoid incising the meniscus, begin the arthrotomy 2 cm above the joint line (see Fig. 9-39).

Posterior Arthrotomy

To inspect the posterior horn of the lateral meniscus, find the lateral head of the gastrocnemius at its origin at the back of the lateral condyle of the femur. Dissect between it and the posterolateral corner of the joint capsule. The lateral superior genicular arteries are in this area; they must be ligated or coagulated.

Note that the popliteus muscle inserts into the femur by way of a tendon that lies inside the

FIG. 9-38. Internervous plane between the *iliotibial band* (superior gluteal nerve) and the *biceps femoris* (sciatic nerve).

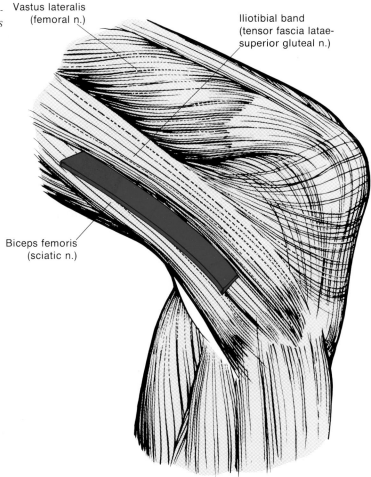

Vastus lateralis (femoral n.)

Iliotibial band (tensor fascia latae-superior gluteal n.)

Biceps femoris (sciatic n.)

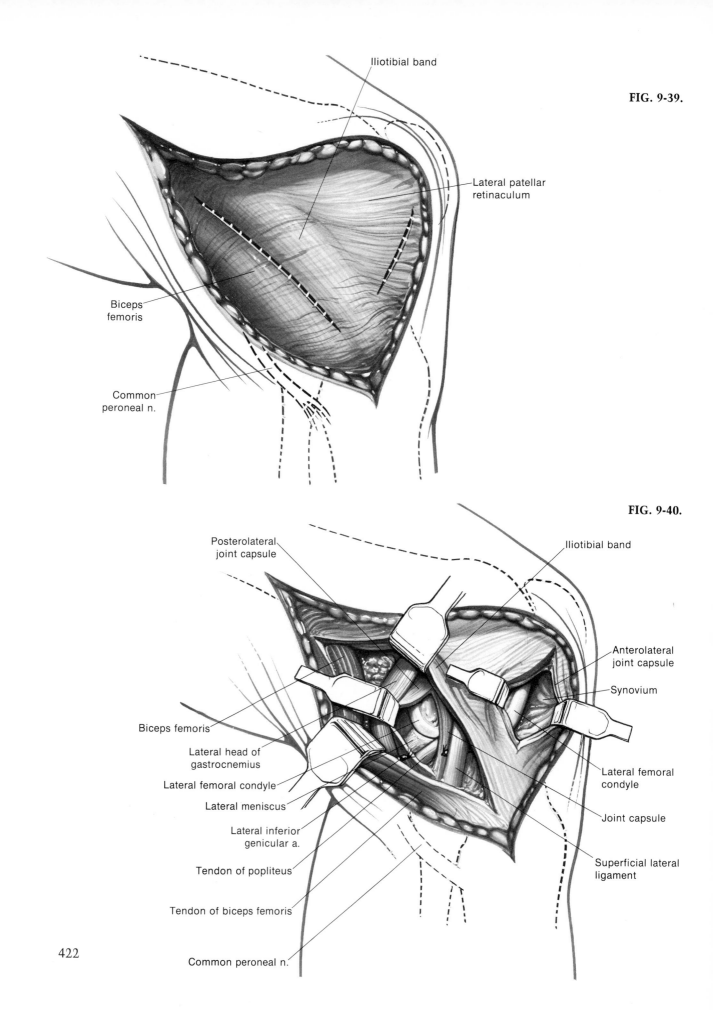

FIG. 9-39.

Iliotibial band

Lateral patellar retinaculum

Biceps femoris

Common peroneal n.

FIG. 9-40.

Posterolateral joint capsule

Iliotibial band

Anterolateral joint capsule

Synovium

Biceps femoris

Lateral head of gastrocnemius

Lateral femoral condyle

Lateral meniscus

Lateral inferior genicular a.

Tendon of popliteus

Tendon of biceps femoris

Lateral femoral condyle

Joint capsule

Superficial lateral ligament

Common peroneal n.

FIG. 9-39. Incise the fascia in the interval between the iliotibial band and the biceps femoris to uncover the superficial lateral (fibular collateral) ligament and the posterior joint complex. Make a separate fascial incision anteriorly to create a lateral parapatellar approach.

FIG. 9-40. Make an incision into the joint capsule anterior to the superficial lateral ligament for a standard anterolateral approach. To enter the posterior portion of the joint, retract the iliotibial band anteriorly and the biceps femoris posteriorly, revealing the superficial lateral ligament and the posterolateral aspect of the joint. Incise the joint capsule posterior to the ligament to reveal the contents of the joint.

joint capsule; the posterolateral corner of the knee may be hidden by the popliteus and its tendon. In cases of trauma, the dissection in this area may already have been done for you.

Make a longitudinal incision in the capsule, starting the arthrotomy well above the joint line to avoid damaging the meniscus or the tendon of the popliteus. An arthrotomy of the posterior half of the joint capsule must be performed carefully to avoid damaging the popliteus tendon, which lies outside the meniscus. The arthrotomy allows you to inspect the posterior half of the lateral compartment behind the superficial lateral ligament (see Fig. 9-40).

DANGERS

Nerves

The **common peroneal nerve** is the structure most at risk during the approach. It lies on the posterior border of the biceps tendon. It must be found early in the approach, as the supporting structures of the lateral side of the knee are being dissected; thereafter, it must be protected, because it is easy to damage. The nerve should be identified proximal to any damage and traced from a normal into an abnormal area (see Fig. 9-41).

Vessels

The **lateral superior genicular artery** runs between the lateral head of the gastrocnemius and the posterolateral capsule and requires ligation for full exposure of that corner of the joint (see Fig. 9-43).

Muscles and Ligaments

The **popliteus tendon** is at risk as it travels within the joint before it attaches to the posterior aspect of the meniscus and the femur. Take care when you open the posterior half of the knee joint capsule to avoid cutting the tendon (see Fig. 9-43).

SPECIAL PROBLEMS

The **lateral meniscus** or its **coronary ligament** may be accidentally incised if arthrotomies are performed too close to the joint line.

HOW TO ENLARGE THE APPROACH

Local Measures

The approach as described gives a complete view of the lateral structures of the knee and cannot be usefully improved.

Extensile Measures

The exposure cannot be usefully extended.

APPLIED SURGICAL ANATOMY OF THE LATERAL SIDE OF THE KNEE

OVERVIEW

The supporting structures on the lateral side of the knee fall into three layers. Because the anatomy can be distorted in pathologic states, a clear understanding of the normal anatomy is required before explorations[17] are carried out.

Outer Layer

The outer layer is continuous with the deep fascia of the thigh (Fig. 9-41). The *iliotibial band,* the aponeurotic tendon of the tensor fasciae latae and gluteus maximus muscles, is a thickening in the deep fascia of the thigh. Its fibers run longitudinally.

The band inserts into a smooth facet on the anterior surface of the lateral condyle of the tibia, known as Gerdy's tubercle. It also sends fibers into the deep fascia of the leg and reinforces the lateral patellar retinaculum. In severe varus injuries to the knee, its insertion may be avulsed. When the knee is in extension, the iliotibial band is anterior to the axis of motion and maintains extension. With the knee flexed to 90°, it moves behind the axis of motion and can act as a flexor.

The *biceps femoris,* a part of the outer layer, is enclosed by the deep fascia like the sartorius on the medial side. (For details of its anatomy, see pp. 379, 385.)

The *lateral patellar retinaculum* is a tough structure derived largely from the fascia covering the vastus lateralis.

Middle Layer

The superficial lateral ligament (fibular collateral ligament) runs from the lateral epicondyle of the femur to the head of the fibula. The lateral inferior genicular vessels run between the ligament and the joint capsule itself. Because the ligament is at-tached to the femoral condyle behind the axis of rotation, it is tight in extension. When the liga-ment is damaged, subsequent functional problems are minimized by the existence of other supporting structures on the lateral side of the knee, especially the iliotibial band (Fig. 9-42).

Deep Layer

The deep layer consists of the true capsule of the knee joint, the fibrous tissue attached just above and below the articular surfaces of the knee. Two other structures run with the capsule:

1. The *popliteus* originates from the popliteal sur-face of the tibia above the soleal line. Its ten-don, which lies within the joint capsule, at-taches to the lateral condyle of the femur and the posterior aspect of the lateral meniscus.

FIG. 9-41. A slightly anterolateral view of the outer layer of the knee. The lateral patellar retinaculum, the biceps femoris, and the iliotibial band constitute the outer layer.

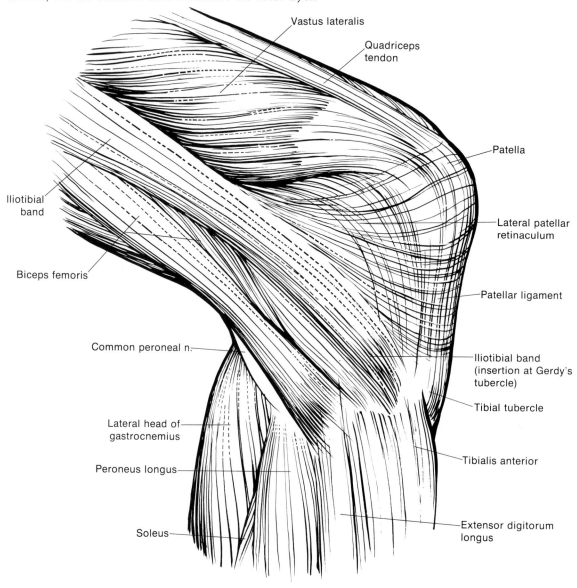

2. The *short lateral ligament* (deep lateral ligament) is a thickening in the true capsule of the knee. The ligament is poorly developed; it runs underneath the superficial lateral (fibular collateral) ligament, from the lateral femoral condyle to the head of the fibula. Unlike the medial ligament, the lateral ligament does not attach to the meniscus. That is why the lateral meniscus can move far more freely than its medial counterpart (see Fig. 9-43).

LANDMARKS AND INCISION

Oblique or longitudinal skin incisions cross the lines of cleavage almost perpendicularly and may result in broad scars.

SUPERFICIAL AND DEEP DISSECTIONS

I. *Approach for Lateral Meniscectomy*
 1. Incise the *superficial* and *deep layers,* cutting the lateral patellar retinaculum (see Fig. 9-42).

FIG. 9-42. The lateral patellar retinaculum, the iliotibial band, and the deep fascia (outer layer) have been excised to reveal the superficial lateral ligament (middle layer) and the joint capsule (deep layer). Note that the lateral inferior genicular artery runs along the joint line between the middle and deep layers.

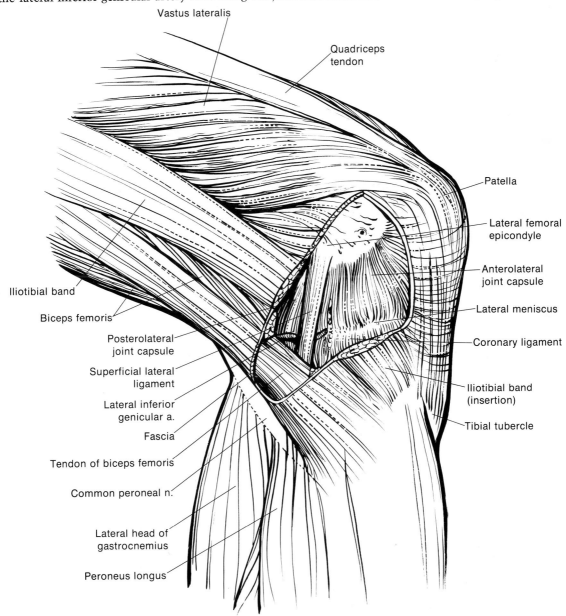

Vastus lateralis

Quadriceps tendon

Patella

Lateral femoral epicondyle

Anterolateral joint capsule

Lateral meniscus

Coronary ligament

Iliotibial band (insertion)

Tibial tubercle

Iliotibial band

Biceps femoris

Posterolateral joint capsule

Superficial lateral ligament

Lateral inferior genicular a.

Fascia

Tendon of biceps femoris

Common peroneal n.

Lateral head of gastrocnemius

Peroneus longus

2. The true capsule of the joint is very thin at this point. Incise it with its synovium to gain access to the joint surface.

II. *Lateral Exposure of the Knee and Its Supporting Structures*

1. Open the *superficial layer* in the plane between the biceps femoris and the iliotibial band (see Fig. 9-42).
2. Incise the joint either in front of or behind the superficial lateral ligament, the lateral side's *middle layer* (Fig. 9-43).
3. Incise the capsule of the joint *(deep layer)* in front of or behind the superficial lateral ligament. Do not damage the tendon of the popliteus, which lies between the outer border of the lateral meniscus and the capsule of the joint (see Fig. 9-43).

FIG. 9-43. A true lateral view of the knee joint. The biceps femoris, iliotibial band, and vastus lateralis have been excised to reveal the deeper layers. The joint capsule has been excised anterior and posterior to the superficial lateral ligament (fibular collateral ligament) to expose the intra-articular structures, notably the popliteus tendon and the lateral meniscus.

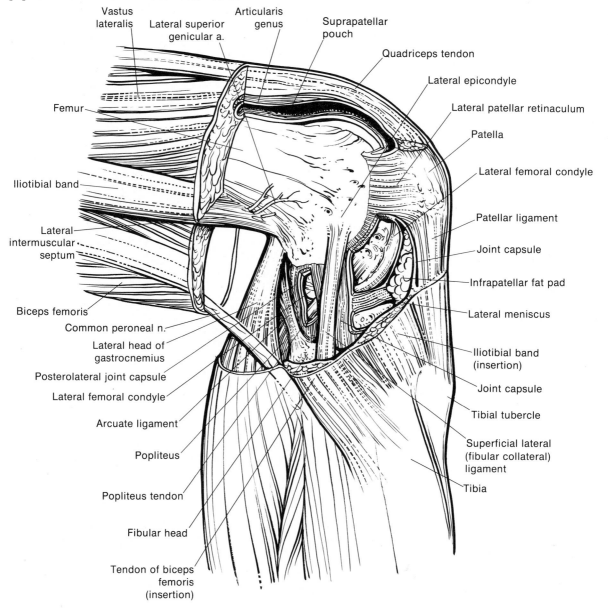

POSTERIOR APPROACH TO THE KNEE

The posterior approach[1,18] is primarily a neurovascular approach. Orthopaedically, it is rarely needed since the medial and lateral approaches each give good access to half the posterior capsule. Its uses include the following:

1. Repair of the neurovascular structures that run behind the knee in cases of trauma
2. Repair of avulsion fractures of the site of attachment of the posterior cruciate ligament to the tibia
3. Recession of gastrocnemius heads in cases of contracture
4. Lengthening of hamstring tendons
5. Excision of Baker's cyst and other popliteal cysts
6. Access to the posterior capsule of the knee

POSITION OF PATIENT.

Place the patient prone on the operating table. Use a tourniquet for all procedures except vascular repairs (Fig. 9-44).

LANDMARKS AND INCISION

Landmarks

Palpate the two heads of the *gastrocnemius muscle* at their origin on the posterior femoral surface just above the medial and lateral condyles. They are not as easy to feel as the hamstring tendons just above them.

Palpate the *semimembranosus and semitendinosus* muscles on the medial border of the popliteal fossa. The semitendinosus feels round; the semimembranosus is deeper and remains muscular to its insertion.

Incision

Use an S-shaped incision. Start laterally over the biceps femoris and bring the incision obliquely across the popliteal fossa. Turn downward over the medial head of the gastrocnemius and run the incision inferiorly into the calf (Fig. 9-45).

INTERNERVOUS PLANE

There is no true internervous plane in this dissection, which exposes the contents of the popliteal fossa by incising the deep fascia over it and by pulling apart the three muscles that form its boundaries.

SUPERFICIAL SURGICAL DISSECTION

Reflect the skin flaps to reveal the *small* (short) saphenous vein as it passes upward just about in the midline of the calf. The vein is easier to identify if the leg is not fully exsanguinated before the tourniquet is applied. Running on the lateral side of the vein is the medial sural cutaneous nerve. You can use the *small* saphenous vein as a guide to the nerve and the nerve, in turn, as a guide to dissecting the popliteal fossa. The nerve, which continues beneath the deep fascia of the calf, is a branch of the tibial nerve (Fig. 9-46; see Fig. 9-49).

Incise the fascia of the popliteal fossa just medial to the small saphenous vein. Trace the medial sural cutaneous nerve proximally back to its source, the tibial nerve. Dissect up to the apex of the popliteal fossa, following the tibial nerve (Fig. 9-47).

The apex of the popliteal fossa is formed by the semimembranosus on the medial side and the biceps femoris on the lateral side. Roughly at the apex, the common peroneal nerve separates from the tibial nerve. Dissect out the common peroneal nerve from proximal to distal as it runs along the posterior border of the biceps femoris (Fig. 9-48; see Fig. 9-51).

Now turn to the popliteal artery and vein, which lie deep and medial to the tibial nerve (Fig. 9-49). The artery has five branches around the knee: two superior, two inferior, and one middle genicular artery. One or more of these branches may have to be ligated if the artery needs to be mobilized (see Fig. 9-52).

The popliteal vein lies medial to the artery as it enters the popliteal fossa from below. Then it

FIG. 9-44. Position of the patient on the operating table for the posterior approach to the femur.

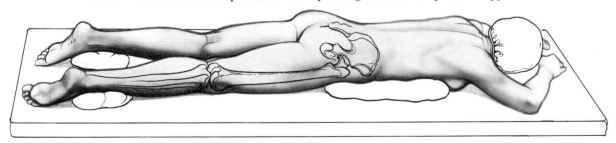

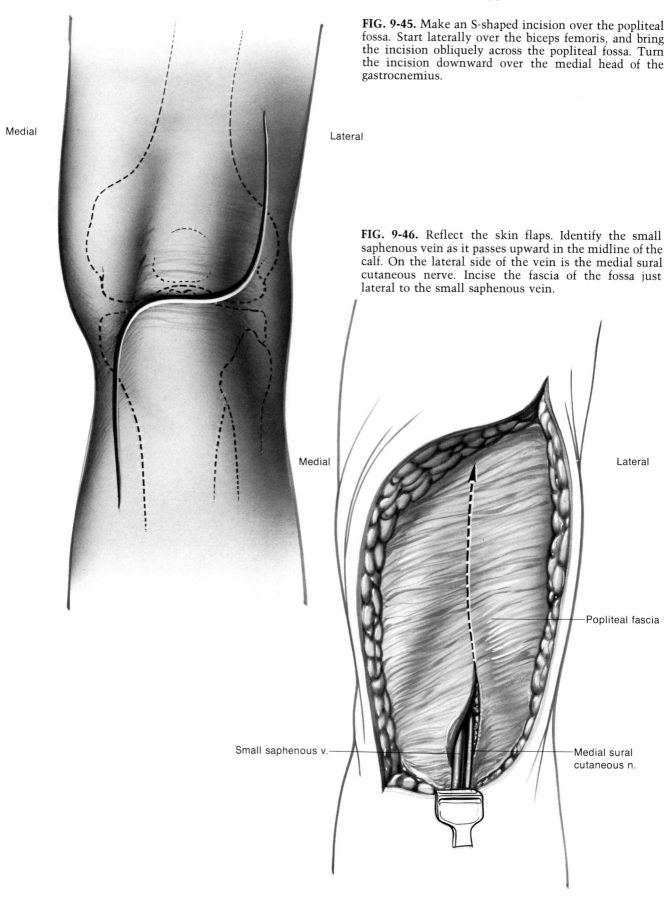

FIG. 9-45. Make an S-shaped incision over the popliteal fossa. Start laterally over the biceps femoris, and bring the incision obliquely across the popliteal fossa. Turn the incision downward over the medial head of the gastrocnemius.

FIG. 9-46. Reflect the skin flaps. Identify the small saphenous vein as it passes upward in the midline of the calf. On the lateral side of the vein is the medial sural cutaneous nerve. Incise the fascia of the fossa just lateral to the small saphenous vein.

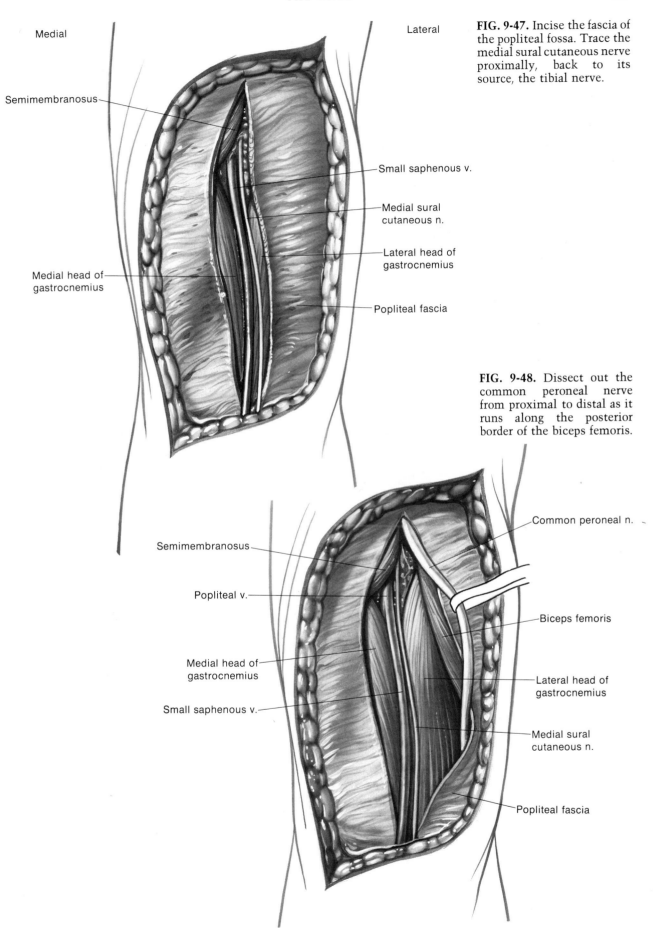

Medial

Lateral

Semimembranosus

Small saphenous v.

Medial sural
cutaneous n.

Lateral head of
gastrocnemius

Medial head of
gastrocnemius

Popliteal fascia

FIG. 9-47. Incise the fascia of the popliteal fossa. Trace the medial sural cutaneous nerve proximally, back to its source, the tibial nerve.

FIG. 9-48. Dissect out the common peroneal nerve from proximal to distal as it runs along the posterior border of the biceps femoris.

Semimembranosus

Common peroneal n.

Popliteal v.

Biceps femoris

Medial head of
gastrocnemius

Lateral head of
gastrocnemius

Small saphenous v.

Medial sural
cutaneous n.

Popliteal fascia

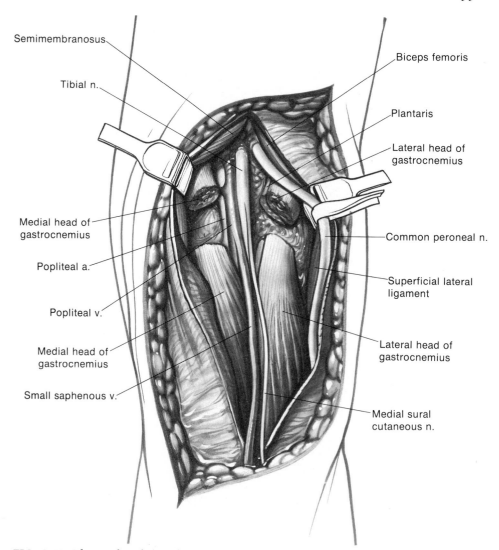

Semimembranosus

Tibial n.

Biceps femoris

Plantaris

Lateral head of gastrocnemius

Medial head of gastrocnemius

Popliteal a.

Common peroneal n.

Popliteal v.

Superficial lateral ligament

Medial head of gastrocnemius

Lateral head of gastrocnemius

Small saphenous v.

Medial sural cutaneous n.

FIG. 9-49. The popliteal vein lies medial to the artery as it enters the popliteal fossa from below. Then it curves, lying directly posterior to the artery while in the fossa.

curves, lying directly posterior to the artery while in the fossa. Above the knee joint, it moves to the posterolateral side of the artery (see Fig. 8-40).

DEEP SURGICAL DISSECTION

Retracting the muscles that form the boundaries of the popliteal fossa exposes various parts of the posterior joint capsule. There are two ways to gain greater access to the joint if you need it:

1. Posteromedial joint capsule. Detach the tendinous origin of the medial head of the gastrocnemius from the back of the femur. Retract the head laterally and inferiorly, pulling the nerves and vessels out of the way to reach the posteromedial corner of the joint.

The exposure is now the same as that achieved by the posterior extension of the medial approach to the knee (Fig. 9-50; see Fig. 9-49).

2. Posterolateral corner of the joint. Detach the origin of the lateral head of the gastrocnemius from the lateral femoral condyle. Develop the interval between it and the biceps femoris, creating the same exposure as the lateral approach to the knee (see Figs. 9-49 and 9-50).

Note that the posterior approach is no better than the lateral and medial approaches in dealing with pathology of the posteromedial and posterolateral corners of the knee joint. It should be used mainly for exploration of structures within the popliteal fossa and for reattachment of the avulsed tibial insertion of the posterior cruciate ligament.

into the back of the calf. It travels roughly along the midline of the calf and penetrates the popliteal fascia before joining the popliteal vein.

2. The *medial sural cutaneous nerve* also runs in the midline of the calf beneath the deep fascia, just lateral to the small saphenous vein. The nerve, a branch of the tibial nerve, supplies varying amounts of skin on the back of the calf.

Knowing the location of these two structures makes it easier to find the tibial nerve (see Fig. 9-51).

The *tibial nerve*, a continuation of the sciatic nerve, is lateral to the popliteal artery as it enters the popliteal fossa. Then, at the midpoint of the fossa, it crosses the artery and lies medial to it as they leave the fossa together. The tibial nerve passes vertically downward in the fossa, giving branches to the plantaris, the gastrocnemius, the soleus, and the popliteus. Its sole cutaneous branch, the sural nerve, is of surgical interest in nerve grafting. The tibial nerve leaves the fossa between the two heads of the gastrocnemius. Tibial nerve palsy affects the plantar flexors of the toes and ankle (Fig. 9-52).

The *common peroneal nerve* slopes downward across the fossa, running laterally toward the medial side of the tendon of the biceps. It disappears into the peroneus longus before winding around the fibula. Its division into deep and superficial peroneal nerves occurs within the substance of the peroneus longus. Common peroneal nerve palsy affects all the extensors and evertors of the foot (see Fig. 9-52) (see Figs. 10-15 and 10-26).

The vascular structures lie more deeply in the fossa. The popliteal artery runs obliquely through the fossa after entering on the medial side of the femur. It lies directly behind the posterior capsule of the knee joint, dividing into its terminal branches, the posterior tibial, anterior tibial, and peroneal arteries, behind the gastrocnemius. In the fossa, it gives off five branches:

The *two superior genicular arteries* encircle the lower end of the femur. The lateral artery requires ligation in the posterolateral approach to the knee. The medial artery requires ligation if the medial head of the gastrocnemius has to be detached from the femur to expose the posteromedial corner of the knee.

The *middle genicular artery* passes forward in the

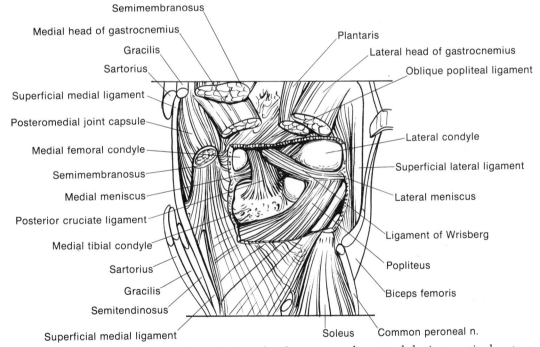

FIG. 9-54. The posterior joint capsule of the knee has been resected to reveal the intra-articular structures of the posterior aspect of the knee, most notably the posterior cruciate ligament and the popliteus.

Popliteus. *Origin.* Popliteal surface of tibia above soleal line. *Insertion.* Lateral epicondyle of femur and posterior aspect of lateral meniscus. *Action.* Rotates femur laterally on tibia. *Nerve supply.* Tibial nerve.

knee and supplies the cruciate ligament. The artery holds its parent trunk firmly to the posterior capsule of the joint. For this reason, it can easily be damaged in traumatic dislocations of the knee or during surgery. It may also be damaged as you dissect out posterior structures in the knee from medial or lateral approaches. To avoid endangering it, flex the knee to allow the joint capsule to fall away from the back of the femur and tibia.

The *two inferior genicular arteries* (medial and lateral) encircle the upper end of the tibia, passing deep to the medial and lateral superficial ligaments. The lateral artery is the most commonly damaged structure during lateral meniscectomy; it runs right at the level of the joint line and is therefore vulnerable in cases in which the meniscus is detached too far laterally (see Fig. 9-52).

The *popliteal vein* lies between the popliteal artery and the tibial nerve. The small saphenous vein pierces the popliteal fascia to enter the popliteal vein within the fossa.

DEEP SURGICAL DISSECTION AND ITS DANGERS

Deep surgical dissection consists in retracting and, sometimes, mobilizing the boundaries of the popliteal fossa. These boundaries are formed by the semimembranosus and semitendinosus (superomedial), the biceps femoris (superolateral), the medial head of gastrocnemius (inferomedial), and the lateral head of gastrocnemius (inferolateral) (see Fig. 9-52). For more information on these muscles, see the pages listed below.

Semimembranosus (pp. 381–387)
Semitendinosus (pp. 381–387)
Biceps femoris (p. 385)
Gastrocnemius (pp. 462–466)

The floor of the popliteal fossa is formed by the *popliteus*, one of the few muscles in the body whose origin is distal to its insertion. The tendon enters the joint by passing through a gap in the posterolateral capsule, beneath the arcuate ligament (Figs. 9-53 and 9-54).

The popliteus unlocks the knee from its fully extended (screw home) position. It also draws the lateral femoral condyle backward on the tibia and pulls the lateral meniscus back, preventing it from being trapped between the tibia and femur. The convex rounded posterior aspect of the lateral tibial plateau allows this movement to take place.

LATERAL APPROACH TO THE DISTAL FEMUR

The lateral approach to the distal femur, known as the "over-the-top" approach, is used in conjunction with the medial parapatellar approach for the repair or reconstruction of the anterior cruciate ligament. (See Medial Parapatellar Approach.) It is, therefore, not used as an isolated incision. The approach exposes the posterior aspect of the intercondylar notch by passing over the top of the posterior aspect of the lateral femoral condyle.

The lateral approach to the distal femur also gives access to the lateral aspect of the lateral femoral condyle so that drill holes can be made in the condyle (if they are needed) for the reattachment of the femoral end of the anterior cruciate ligament.

FIG. 9-55. Position for the lateral approach to the distal femur.

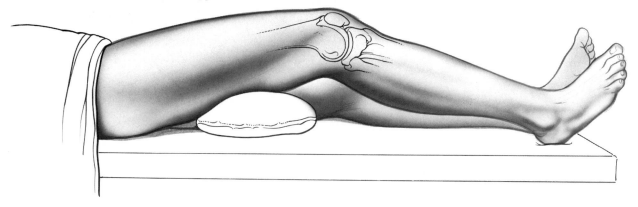

POSITION OF PATIENT

Place the patient supine on the table with a bolster under the thigh so that the knee rests in 30° of flexion. Place a tourniquet high on the patient's thigh and exsanguinate the leg with the use of a compression bandage or by prolonged elevation before inflating a tourniquet (Fig. 9-55).

LANDMARKS AND INCISION

Landmarks

Palpate the posterior lateral margin of the *lateral femoral condyle* as it flares out from the shaft of the femur.

Note the intersection between the *iliotibial band* and the *biceps femoris.*

Incision

Make a 10-cm long incision parallel to and over the indentation between the biceps femoris and the iliotibial band. Distally, the incision ends at the flare of the femoral condyle (Fig. 9-56).

INTERNERVOUS PLANE

The dissection exploits the internervous plane between the *vastus lateralis muscle* (supplied by the femoral nerve) and the *biceps femoris* (supplied by the sciatic nerve) (see Fig. 9-38).

SUPERFICIAL SURGICAL DISSECTION

Incise the iliotibial band just anterior to the lateral intermuscular septum, in line with the skin incision. The incision is slightly anterior to the skin incision itself (Fig. 9-57).

DEEP SURGICAL DISSECTION

Identify the vastus lateralis anterior to the intermuscular septum and retract it anteriorly and medially. Below the muscle lies the lateral superior genicular artery; it must be ligated (Figs. 9-58 and 9-59). With a cautery, incise the periosteum at the junction of the shaft and flare of the femur. Pass a small clamp or a small Cobb elevator behind the posterolateral flare of the lateral femoral condyle,

FIG. 9-56. Make a 10-cm long incision parallel to and over the indentation between the biceps femoris and the iliotibial band.

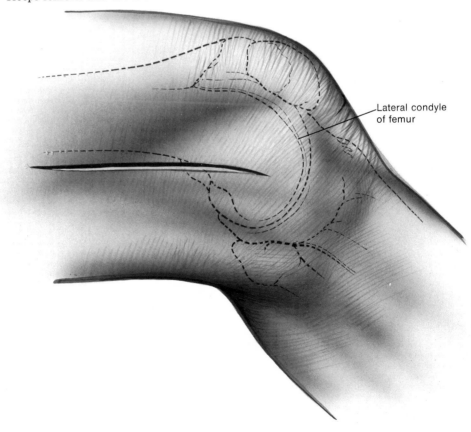

Lateral condyle of femur

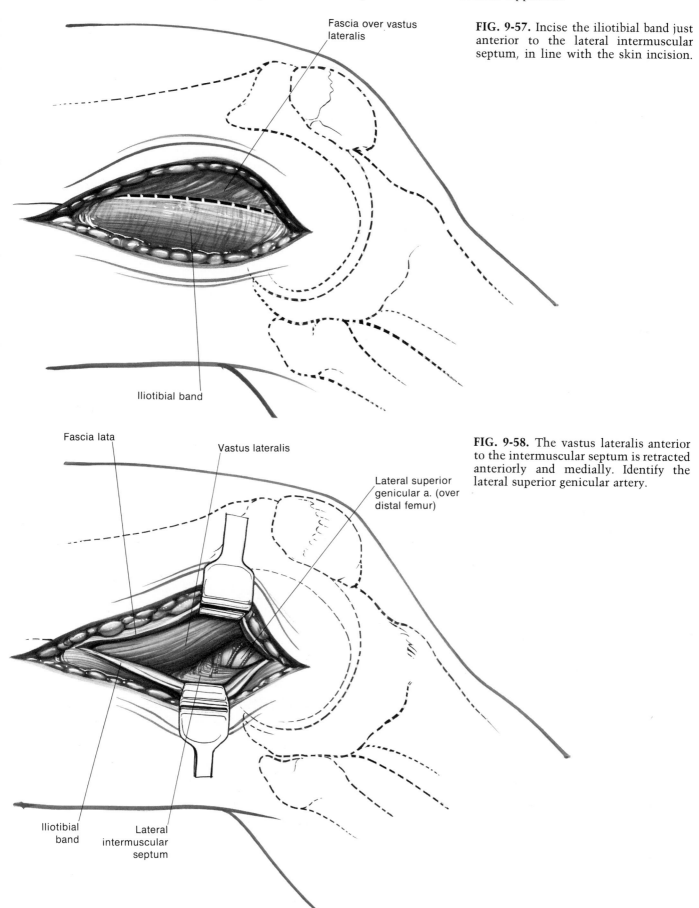

Fascia over vastus lateralis

FIG. 9-57. Incise the iliotibial band just anterior to the lateral intermuscular septum, in line with the skin incision.

Iliotibial band

Fascia lata

Vastus lateralis

Lateral superior genicular a. (over distal femur)

FIG. 9-58. The vastus lateralis anterior to the intermuscular septum is retracted anteriorly and medially. Identify the lateral superior genicular artery.

Iliotibial band

Lateral intermuscular septum

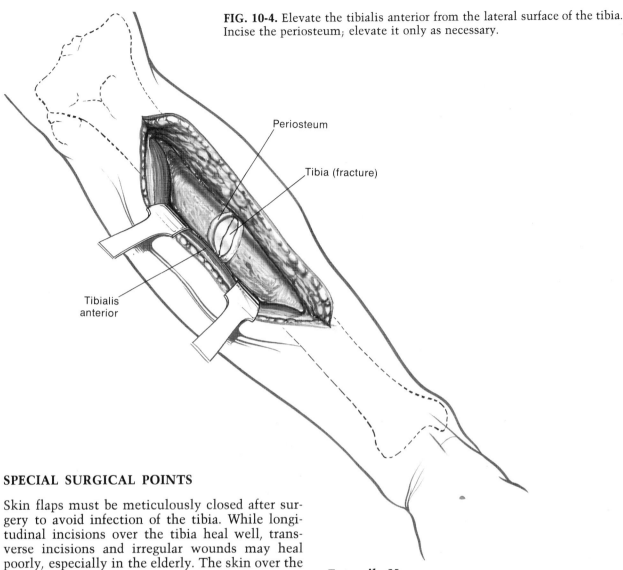

FIG. 10-4. Elevate the tibialis anterior from the lateral surface of the tibia. Incise the periosteum; elevate it only as necessary.

Periosteum

Tibia (fracture)

Tibialis anterior

SPECIAL SURGICAL POINTS

Skin flaps must be meticulously closed after surgery to avoid infection of the tibia. While longitudinal incisions over the tibia heal well, transverse incisions and irregular wounds may heal poorly, especially in the elderly. The skin over the lower third of the tibia is very thin; wounds in that area heal badly, especially in patients with chronic venous insufficiency.

HOW TO ENLARGE THE APPROACH

Local Measures

The extent of the exposure is determined by the size of the skin incision; the whole subcutaneous surface of the tibia may be exposed, if necessary.

To reach the posterior surface of the tibia from an anterior approach, continue the subperiosteal dissection posteriorly around the medial border. Proximally, lift the flexor digitorum longus off the posterior surface of the tibia subperiosteally. Distally, lift off the tibialis posterior muscle. This procedure exposes the posterior surface of the bone but does not offer as full an exposure as the posterolateral approach.

Extensile Measures

PROXIMAL EXTENSION. To extend the approach proximally, continue the skin incision along the medial side of the patella. Deepen the incision through the medial patellar retinaculum to gain access to the knee joint and the patella. (For details, see Chapter 9, p. 390.) Alternatively, extend the wound proximally along the lateral side of the patella. Deepen that wound through the lateral patellar retinaculum to gain access to the lateral compartment of the knee. (For details, see Chapter 9, p. 415.)

DISTAL EXTENSION. To extend the approach distally, curve the incision over the medial side of the hind part of the foot. Deepening the wound gives access to all the structures that pass behind the medial malleolus. Continue the incision onto the mid part and fore part of the foot. (For details, see Chapter 11, pp. 474, 480.)

POSTEROLATERAL APPROACH TO THE TIBIA

The posterolateral approach[4] is used to expose the middle two thirds of the tibia when the skin over the subcutaneous surface is badly scarred or infected. It is a technically demanding operation. The approach is suitable for the following:

1. Internal fixation of fractures
2. Treatment of delayed union or nonunion[5] fractures, including bone grafting

The approach also permits exposure of the middle of the posterior aspect of the fibula.

POSITION OF PATIENT

Place the patient on his side, with the affected leg uppermost. Protect the bony prominences of the bottom leg to avoid pressure sores. Exsanguinate the limb by elevating it for 5 minutes, and then apply a tourniquet (Fig. 10-5).

LANDMARKS AND INCISION

Landmark

The lateral border of the *gastrocnemius* muscle is easy to palpate in the calf.

Incision

Make a longitudinal incision over the lateral border of the gastrocnemius. The length of the incision depends on the length of bone that must be exposed (Fig. 10-6).

INTERNERVOUS PLANE

The internervous plane lies between the *gastrocnemius, soleus, and flexor hallucis longus muscles* (all supplied by the tibial nerve) and the *peroneal muscles* (supplied by the superficial peroneal nerve)—between the posterior and lateral muscular compartments (Fig. 10-7).

SUPERFICIAL SURGICAL DISSECTION

Reflect the skin flaps, taking care not to damage the short saphenous vein, which runs up the posterolateral aspect of the leg from behind the lateral malleolus. Incise the fascia in line with the incision and find the plane between the lateral head of the gastrocnemius and the soleus posteriorly and the peroneus brevis and longus anteriorly. Muscular branches of the peroneal artery

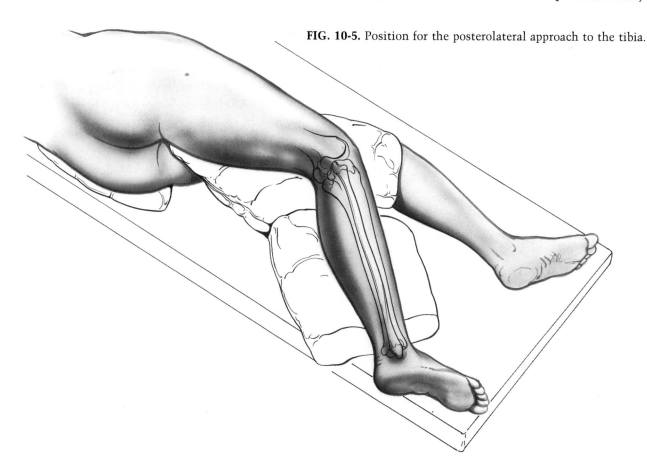

FIG. 10-5. Position for the posterolateral approach to the tibia.

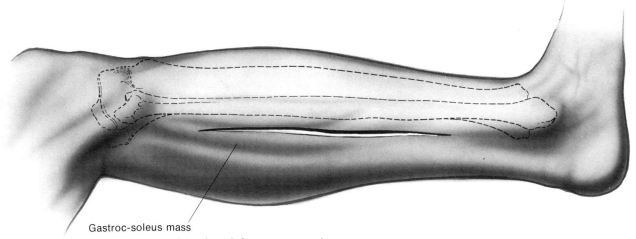

Gastroc-soleus mass

FIG. 10-6. Incision of the lateral border of the gastrocnemius.

FIG. 10-7. The internervous plane lies between the *gastrocnemius, soleus, and flexor hallucis longus muscles* (tibial nerve) and the *peroneal muscles* (superficial peroneal nerve).

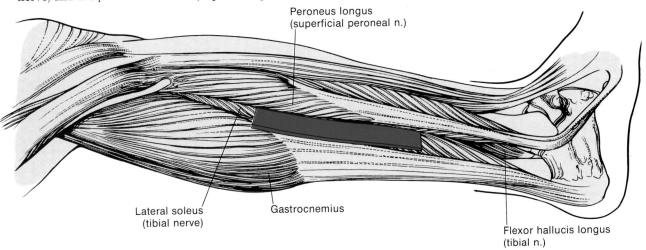

Peroneus longus
(superficial peroneal n.)

Lateral soleus
(tibial nerve)

Gastrocnemius

Flexor hallucis longus
(tibial n.)

lie with the peroneus brevis in the proximal part of the incision and may have to be ligated (Fig. 10-8).

Find the lateral border of the soleus and retract it with the gastrocnemius medially and posteriorly; underneath, arising from the posterior surface of the fibula, is the flexor hallucis longus (Fig. 10-9 and *cross section*).

DEEP SURGICAL DISSECTION

Detach the lower part of the origin of the soleus from the fibula and retract it posteriorly and medially. Detach the flexor hallucis longus from its origin on the fibula and retract it posteriorly and medially (Fig. 10-10 and *cross section*; see Fig. 10-9). Continue dissecting medially across the interosseous membrane, detaching those fibers of the tibialis posterior that arise from it.

The posterior tibial artery and tibial nerve are posterior to the dissection, separated from it by the bulk of the tibialis posterior and the flexor hallucis longus (Fig. 10-11 and *cross section*). Follow the interosseous membrane to the lateral border of the tibia, detaching the muscles that arise from its posterior surface subperiosteally, and expose its posterior surface (Fig. 10-12 and *cross section*).

DANGERS

Vessels

The **small (short) saphenous vein** may be damaged when you mobilize the skin flaps. While you should try to preserve the vein, you may ligate it, if necessary, without impairing venous return from the leg.

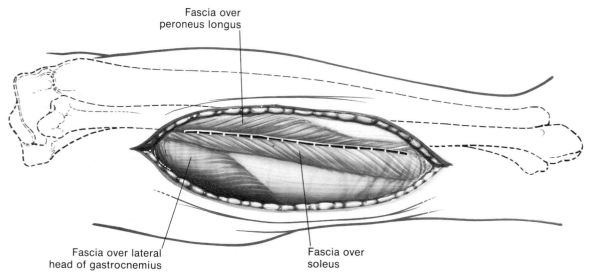

Fascia over
peroneus longus

Fascia over lateral
head of gastrocnemius

Fascia over
soleus

FIG. 10-8. Reflect the skin flaps. Incise the fascia in line with the incision. Find the plane between the lateral head of the gastrocnemius and soleus (posteriorly) and the peroneus brevis and longus (anteriorly).

Branches of the **peroneal artery** cross the intermuscular plane between the gastrocnemius and the peroneus brevis. They should be ligated or coagulated to reduce postoperative bleeding (see Fig. 10-23).

The **posterior tibial artery** and tibial nerve are safe as long as you stay on the interosseous membrane and do not wander into a plane posterior to the flexor hallucis longus and tibialis posterior (see Fig. 10-23).

HOW TO ENLARGE THE APPROACH

Extensile Measures

PROXIMAL EXTENSION. The approach cannot be extended into the proximal fourth of the tibia. There, the back of the tibia is covered by the popliteus muscle and the more superficial posterior tibial artery and tibial nerve, making safe dissection impossible.

DISTAL EXTENSION. The approach can be made continuous with the posterior approach to the ankle if you extend the skin incision distally between the posterior aspect of the lateral malleolus and the tendon of Achilles. (For details, see pp. 484–492.)

FIG. 10-9. Detach the origin of the soleus from the fibula and retract it posteriorly and medially along with the gastrocnemius. Retract the peroneal muscles anteriorly. Detach the flexor hallucis longus from its origin on the fibula. *(Cross section)* Develop the plane between the gastroc-soleus group posteriorly and the peroneal muscles anteriorly. Note the flexor hallucis longus on the posterior surface of the fibula.

FIG. 10-10. Detach the flexor hallucis longus from its origin on the fibula and retract it posteriorly and medially. Continue dissecting posteriorly, staying on the posterior surface of the fibula. *(Cross section)* Detach the flexor hallucis longus from its origin on the fibula, staying close to the bone. Retract the muscle medially.

INTERNERVOUS PLANE

The internervous plane lies between the *peroneal muscles*, supplied by the superficial peroneal nerve, and the *flexor muscles*, supplied by the tibial nerve (see Fig. 10-7).

SUPERFICIAL SURGICAL DISSECTION

To expose the fibular head and neck, begin proximally by incising the deep fascia in line with the incision, taking great care not to cut the underlying common peroneal nerve. Find the posterior border of the biceps femoris tendon as it sweeps down past the knee before inserting into the head of the fibula. Identify and isolate the common peroneal nerve in its course behind the biceps tendon; trace it as it winds around the fibular neck (Fig. 10-14*A* and *B*). Mobilize the nerve from the groove on the back of the neck by cutting the fibers of the peroneus longus that cover the nerve and gently pulling the nerve forward over the fibular head with a strip of corrugated rubber drain. Identify and preserve all branches of the nerve (Fig. 10-15).

Develop a plane between the peroneal and the soleus; with the common peroneal nerve retracted anteriorly, incise the periosteum of the fibula longitudinally in line with this plane of cleavage. Continue the incision down to bone (Fig. 10-16).

DEEP SURGICAL DISSECTION

Strip the muscles off the fibula by dissection. All muscles that originate from the fibula have fibers that run distally toward the foot and ankle. Therefore, to strip them off cleanly, you must elevate them from distal to proximal. Most muscles originate from periosteum or fascia; they can be stripped. Muscles attached directly to bone are difficult to strip; they usually must be cut (Fig. 10-17 and *cross section*).

The other structure attached to the fibula, the interosseous membrane, has fibers that run obliquely upward. To complete the dissection, strip the interosseous membrane subperiosteally from proximal to distal (Fig. 10-18 and *cross section*).

DANGERS

Nerves

The **common peroneal nerve** is vulnerable as it winds around the neck of the fibula. The key to preserving the nerve is to identify it proximally as it lies on the posterior border of the biceps femoris. It then can be safely traced through the peroneal muscle mass and retracted. The dorsal cutaneous branch of the superficial peroneal nerve is susceptible to injury at the junction of the distal and middle thirds of the fibula; if it is damaged, it causes numbness on the dorsum of the foot (see Fig. 10-26).

Vessels

Terminal branches of the **peroneal artery** lie close to the deep surface of the lateral malleolus. To avoid damaging them, you must keep the dissection subperiosteal (see Fig. 10-23).

The **small (short) saphenous vein** may be damaged; you may ligate it if necessary.

FIG. 10-16. Develop the intermuscular plane between the peroneal muscles and the soleus down the lateral edge of the fibula. Strip the flexor muscles from the posterior aspect of the fibula, going from distal to proximal.

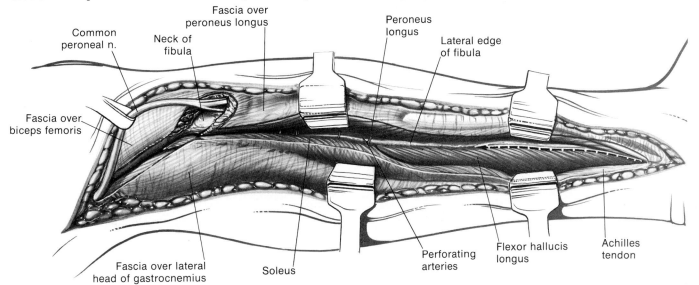

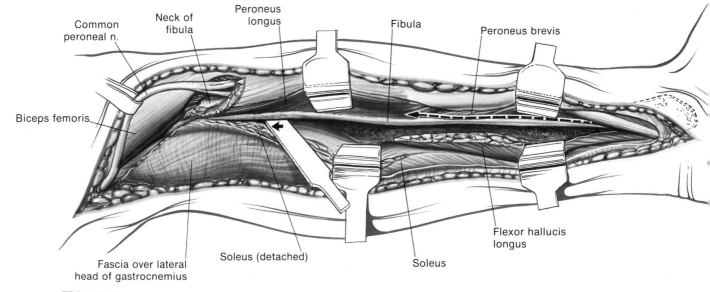

FIG. 10-17.

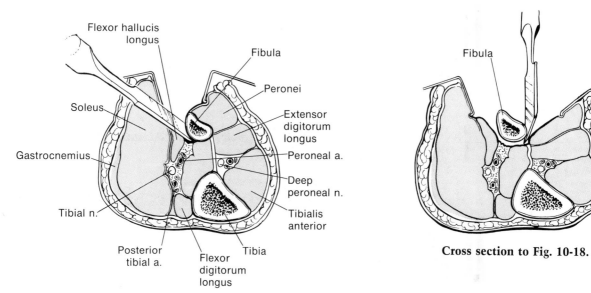

Cross section to Fig. 10-17.

Cross section to Fig. 10-18.

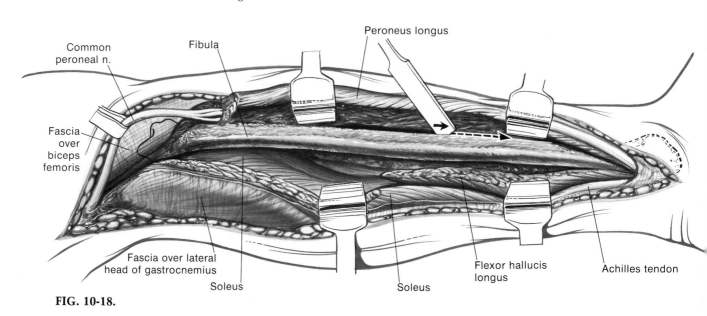

FIG. 10-18.

◄ **FIG. 10-17.** Strip the flexor hallucis longus and the soleus from the posterior aspect of the fibula and strip the peroneal muscles from the anterior surface of the fibula from distal to proximal. *(Cross section)* Strip the flexor muscles from the posterior aspect of the fibula. Avoid neurovascular structures by staying close to the bone.

◄ **FIG. 10-18.** Retract the peroneal muscles anteriorly. Strip the interosseous membrane from the anterior border of the fibula from proximal to distal. *(Cross section)* Strip the muscles from the anterior surface of the fibula and the interosseous membrane from its fibular attachment from proximal to distal.

HOW TO ENLARGE THE APPROACH

Local Measures

The exposure described allows exposure of the entire bone.

Extensile Measures

DISTAL EXTENSION. Extend the skin incision distally by curving it over the lateral side of the tarsus. To gain access to the sinus tarsi and the talocalcaneal, talonavicular, and calcaneocuboid joints, reflect the underlying extensor digitorum brevis muscle. This extension is frequently used on lateral operations of the leg and foot (see pp. 499–503).

APPLIED SURGICAL ANATOMY OF THE LEG

OVERVIEW

The tibia and fibula are very different bones. The tibia has a large subcutaneous surface that allows access to the bone along its entire length; the fibula is almost completely enclosed in muscle. Only at its proximal end and in the lower third of the bone does the fibula develop a subcutaneous surface, which terminates in the lateral malleolus. For this reason, operations on most of the fibula almost always involve extensive stripping of muscle off bone. In addition, the tibia has no major neurovascular structures running directly on it other than its nutrient artery; the fibula has close ties to the common peroneal nerve and its branches.

The deep fascia of the leg is a tough, fibrous, unyielding structure that encloses the calf muscles. Where the bones become subcutaneous, the fascia is usually attached to the border of the bone.

Two intermuscular septa, one anterior and one posterior, pass from the deep surface of the encircling fascia to the fibula and enclose the peroneal or lateral compartment of the leg.

Three separate muscular compartments exist in the lower leg (Fig. 10-19).

Anterior (Extensor) Compartment

The anterior compartment contains the extensor muscles of the foot and ankle. Its medial boundary is the lateral (extensor) surface of the tibia, and its lateral boundary is the extensor surface of the fibula and anterior intermuscular septum. The anterior compartment is enclosed by the deep fascia of the leg. The deep peroneal nerve supplies all the muscles in the compartment. The compartment's artery is the anterior tibial artery.

Lateral (Peroneal) Compartment

The peroneal compartment is bounded by the anterior intermuscular septum in front, by the posterior intermuscular septum behind, and by the fibula medially. It contains the peroneal muscles, the evertors of the foot. The superficial peroneal nerve supplies all the muscles in the compartment. No artery runs in it; its muscles receive their supply from several branches of the peroneal artery.

Posterior (Flexor) Compartment

The flexor compartment contains the flexors of the foot and ankle. The compartment is separated from the other compartments by a fibro-osseous complex: laterally, from the peroneal compartment, by the posterior intermuscular septum and the posterior medial surface of the fibula; anteriorly, from the extensor compartment, by the interosseous membrane and the posterior (flexor) surface of the tibia. The tibial nerve innervates all the muscles in the compartment; the posterior tibial artery supplies them with blood. The peroneal artery also runs in this compartment and forms part of the blood supply of the muscles.

The flexor compartment consists of two groups of muscles, superficial (gastrocnemius, soleus, plantaris) and deep (tibialis posterior, flexor digitorum longus, flexor hallucis longus), separated by a fascial layer.

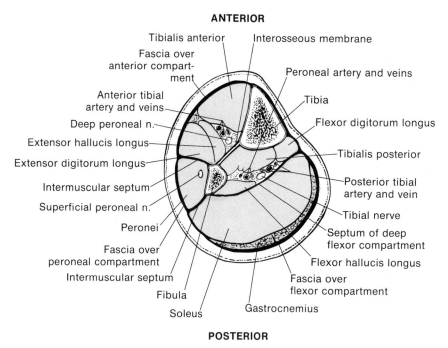

ANTERIOR

Tibialis anterior Interosseous membrane

Fascia over anterior compart-ment

Anterior tibial artery and veins

Deep peroneal n.

Extensor hallucis longus

Extensor digitorum longus

Intermuscular septum

Superficial peroneal n.

Peronei

Fascia over peroneal compartment

Intermuscular septum

Fibula

Soleus

Peroneal artery and veins

Tibia

Flexor digitorum longus

Tibialis posterior

Posterior tibial artery and vein

Tibial nerve

Septum of deep flexor compartment

Flexor hallucis longus

Fascia over flexor compartment

Gastrocnemius

POSTERIOR

FIG. 10-19. The fibro-osseous compartments of the leg.

Anterior Approach to the Tibia

LANDMARKS AND INCISION

Landmark

For the surgeon, the *subcutaneous surface of the tibia* is the most accessible bit of bone in the body. Unfortunately, this ease of access makes the bone attractive as a source of grafts. The procedure weakens the bone, something that is reflected in a high incidence of subsequent fractures.

Incision

The longitudinal incision roughly parallels the lines of cleavage in the skin. The resultant scar is not unduly prominent but is often visible in women because of its position.

SUPERFICIAL SURGICAL DISSECTION

The *periosteum of the tibia* is a thick fibrous membrane that easily can be peeled off the bone, especially in children. Only 10% of the blood supply of the bone comes from the periosteum; the remaining 90% comes from medullary vessels. Therefore, the periosteum can be elevated off a normal bone without a significant impairment of its blood supply. In cases of fracture, however, soft tissue attachments may form the only remaining blood supply to isolated bone fragments and must be preserved.

The *long saphenous vein* is the longest superficial vein in the body. It originates just distal and anterior to the medial malleolus and continues proximally on the medial side of the leg superficial to the fascia. It may be ligated if necessary.

DEEP SURGICAL DISSECTION

The *tibialis anterior* is the only muscle to arise from the tibia in the anterior compartment (Fig. 10-20). The muscle may be partially avulsed from the tibia in joggers and other athletes and is one of the causes of shin splints. The pathology of the complaint is, however, unclear. Some believe that it is caused by stress fractures of the tibia itself; others contend that it represents a compartment syndrome.[10]

The *common peroneal nerve* runs over the neck of the fibula in the substance of the peroneus longus and divides into deep and superficial branches (Fig. 10-21).

The *deep peroneal nerve* continues to wind around the fibular neck deep to the extensor digitorum longus before reaching the anterior surface of the interosseous membrane. It runs down the leg on the interosseous membrane between the tibialis anterior and the extensor hallucis longus, supplying all the muscles of the extensor portion of the leg (see Fig. 10-21).

The *superficial peroneal nerve* runs down the peroneal compartment of the leg, supplying the peroneus longus and brevis. Its dorsal cutaneous branch supplies the skin on the dorsum of the foot (see Fig. 10-21).

The *anterior tibial artery* is a branch of the popliteal artery. It reaches the anterior portion of the leg by passing above the interosseous mem-

FIG. 10-20. The superficial structures of the anterior compartment of the leg.

Tibialis Anterior. *Origin.* Lateral condyle of tibia, upper two thirds of lateral surface of tibia, interosseous membrane, deep fascia, lateral intermuscular septum. *Insertion.* Medial cuneiform and base of first metatarsal. *Action.* Dorsiflexor and invertor of foot. *Nerve supply.* Deep peroneal nerve.

Extensor Hallucis Longus. *Origin.* Middle half of anterior surface of fibula and interosseous membrane. *Insertion.* Base of distal phalanx of hallux. *Action.* Extensor of hallux and ankle. *Nerve supply.* Deep peroneal nerve.

Extensor Digitorum Longus. *Origin.* Upper three fourths of anterior surface of fibula, small area of tibia adjacent to superior tibiofibular joint, and interosseous membrane. *Insertion.* Via extensor hoods to middle and distal phalanges of lateral four toes. *Action.* Extensor of toes and of ankle. *Nerve supply.* Deep peroneal nerve.

Peroneus Tertius. *Origin.* Lower third of anterior surface of fibula. *Insertion.* Base of fifth metatarsal. *Action.* Evertor and dorsiflexor of foot. *Nerve supply.* Deep peroneal nerve.

---

brane. It lies so close to the fibula that its venae comitantes often leave a notch in the bone large enough to be visible on radiographs, a relationship that must be respected when the fibular head is excised. The artery runs with the deep peroneal nerve on the interosseous membrane; it continues in the foot as the dorsalis pedis artery (see Fig. 10-21).

Three other muscles, the extensor hallucis longus, the extensor digitorum longus, and the peroneus tertius, also occupy the anterior compartment of the leg. They are not involved in the anterior approach to the tibia but are a part of the approach to the anterior compartment and may be seen during the exploration of wounds caused by open tibial fractures. Together with the tibialis anterior, they are implicated in the anterior compartment syndrome (see Fig. 10-21).

Posterolateral Approach to the Tibia

LANDMARKS AND INCISION

Incision

The longitudinal incision almost parallels the lines of cleavage in the skin, and the resultant scar is not unduly broad. Cosmesis is rarely a problem during this exposure; it is reserved largely for cases in which the skin on the anterior aspect of the tibia is unsuitable for surgery.

SUPERFICIAL SURGICAL DISSECTION

The superficial surgical dissection consists in finding the plane that separates the gastrocnemius

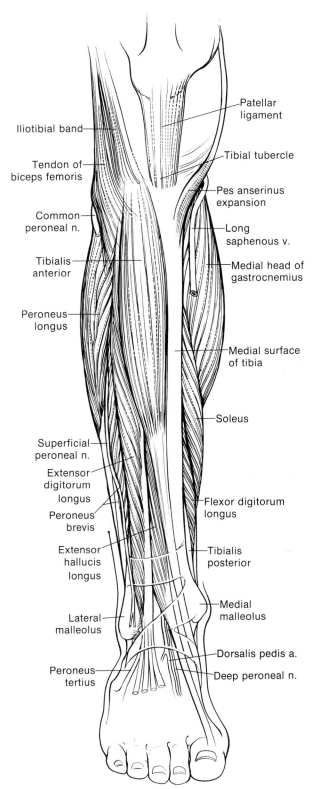

FIG. 10-20.

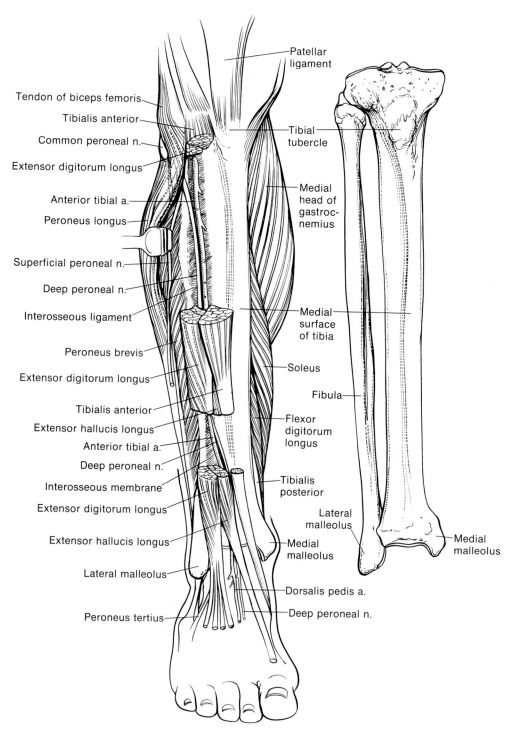

FIG. 10-21. Muscles of the anterior compartment have been resected to reveal the anterior surface of the tibia, the neurovascular structures, the interosseous membrane, and the anterior surface of the fibula.

and soleus from the peroneus brevis (see Fig. 10-25).

The fibers of the *gastrocnemius* are generally arranged longitudinally, giving the muscle the ability to contract a considerable distance at the expense of muscle strength. The muscle crosses two joints. During quiet walking, plantar flexion of the ankle is carried out largely by the powerful soleus muscle, which crosses only one joint. The gastrocnemius is capable of acting as a fast plantar flexor of the ankle, but only if the soleus provides power to overcome the inertia of the body weight. The gastrocnemius, therefore, comes into play mainly during running and jumping.

The major surgical importance of the *soleus* lies in the numerous plexus of small veins that it contains. This multipennate muscle is one of the major pumps involved in venous return from the limb; lack of muscular action, for example, following surgery or fractures, may lead to venous stasis and thrombosis.

The *peroneus brevis* tendon, which grooves the back of the lateral malleolus, is useful in reconstruction of the lateral side of the ankle. On occasion, the peroneus brevis may avulse the styloid process of the fifth metatarsal in association with inversion injuries of the ankle (Figs. 10-22 and 10-25).

DEEP SURGICAL DISSECTION

Deep surgical dissection consists in detaching the flexor hallucis longus from the fibula and the tibialis posterior from the interosseous membrane. Some fibers of the flexor digitorum longus must also be reflected off the posterior surface of the tibia to permit access to that bone.

Generally, the dissection is carried out subperiosteally. Nevertheless, at those points where muscle actually originates from bone, it must be detached by sharp dissection, because a subperiosteal plane cannot be developed (Figs. 10-23 and 10-24).

The *flexor hallucis longus* helps support the longitudinal arch of the foot. In the sole of the foot, it sends slips to the flexors of the second and third toes. It is muscular down to the level of the ankle joint, a characteristic that makes it identifiable at that level.

DANGERS

Nerves and Vessels

The posterior tibial artery and the tibial nerve lie superficial (posterior) to the plane of dissection; they may be damaged if you stray out of plane.

The **posterior tibial artery,** a branch of the popliteal artery, runs under the fibrous arch of the soleus. Its major branch in the calf is the peroneal artery.

The **tibial nerve,** the medial portion of the sciatic nerve, enters the calf deep under the fibrous arch of the soleus. It sends branches to all the muscles of the flexor compartment. Passing behind the medial malleolus, it divides into three branches: a calcaneal branch, a small lateral plantar nerve, and, finally, a larger medial plantar nerve (see Fig. 10-23).

Approach to the Fibula

LANDMARKS AND INCISION

Landmarks

The head and lower end of the *fibula* are palpable. The deep peroneal nerve can be rolled against the fibular neck. The nerve is vulnerable to direct pressure from bandaging, the upper end of a cast, or a bed; it may also be damaged by a careless skin incision. The shaft of the fibula is enclosed in muscles and is palpable only as a resistance felt on the lateral side of the leg.

Incision

The longitudinal incision closely parallels the line of cleavage in the skin, and the resultant scar is not broad and unsightly. As is true for the tibia, incisions made directly over the lower and upper ends of the bone should be closed with special care to ensure sound primary healing.

SUPERFICIAL SURGICAL DISSECTION

Superficial surgical dissection consists in mobilizing the common peroneal nerve as it winds around the neck of the fibula and developing a plane between the peronei and the soleus (see Fig. 10-25).

The *common peroneal nerve* is the lateral portion of the tibial nerve; it is palpable at the neck of the fibula (Fig. 10-26).

DEEP SURGICAL DISSECTION

The deep surgical dissection consists in stripping off those muscles that originate from the fibula: the peroneus longus and peroneus brevis (lateral compartment); the extensor digitorum longus, peroneus tertius, and extensor hallucis longus (anterior compartment); and the flexor digitorum longus, flexor hallucis longus, and soleus (posterior compartment) (see Figs. 10-21 and 10-26).

The *peroneal artery* arises from the posterior tibial artery soon after it leaves the popliteal artery. Relatively small, it runs through the deep

FIG. 10-22. The superficial structures of the posterolateral aspect of the leg. ▶

Gastrocnemius. *Origin.* Medial head from medial condyle and popliteal surface of femur. Lateral head from lateral surface of lateral femoral condyle. Middle third of posterior aspect. *Insertion.* Calcaneus. Into Achilles tendon with soleus and plantaris muscles. Achilles tendon then inserts into calcaneus. *Action.* Plantar flexor of foot. *Nerve supply.* Tibial nerve.

Soleus. *Origin.* Posterior aspect of upper third of fibula, soleal line on tibia, fibrous arch between tibia and fibula. *Insertion.* Middle third of posterior aspect of calcaneus. (Common tendon with gastrocnemius.) *Action.* Plantar flexor of foot. *Nerve supply.* Tibial nerve.

FIG. 10-23. The gastrocnemius and the soleus have been resected to reveal the deep flexor ▶ compartment and the neurovascular structures.

Flexor Hallucis Longus. *Origin.* Lower two thirds of posterior surface fibula, interosseous membrane. *Insertion.* Base of distal phalanx of hallux. *Action.* Flexor of hallux and plantar flexor of foot. *Nerve supply.* Tibial nerve.

Flexor Digitorum Longus. *Origin.* Posterior surface of middle half of tibia and fascia covering tibialis posterior. *Insertion.* Distal phalanges of lateral four toes. *Action.* Flexor of toes and dorsiflexor of foot. *Nerve supply.* Tibial nerve.

flexor compartment of the leg, close to the fibula. Its branches wind around the fibula to supply the peroneus longus. The artery is close to the medial surface of the lower end of the fibula and may be damaged during operations on that part of the bone (see Fig. 10-23).

SPECIAL ANATOMICAL POINTS

Compartment Syndromes

The muscles of the leg are enclosed in tight fibro-osseous compartments. The fascial layers are tough and unyielding, and swelling within a particular compartment rapidly increases pressure. Pressure, in turn, leads to venous stasis, still more intercompartmental pressure, and, eventually, arterial ischemia. Increasing pressure after frac-

tures most commonly occurs in the anterior compartment, even when the fracture is minor and undisplaced, possibly because the fascia is so tight.

The fascial layers define four distinct muscle compartments: anterior (extensor), lateral (peroneal), superficial posterior (flexor), and deep posterior (flexor). All four can be affected by swelling, producing four distinct potential compartment syndromes. Fractures in this area may cause swelling in more than one compartment (see Fig. 10-19).

The compartment most commonly affected is the anterior compartment. It can be decompressed by incising the deep fascia that covers it along its entire length.

All compartments of the leg may be decompressed by excision of the fibula.

ANTERIOR APPROACH TO THE ANKLE

The anterior approach[1] provides an excellent exposure of the ankle joint for arthrodesis. The decision as to whether to use this approach—rather than the lateral transfibular approach, the medial transmalleolar approach, or the posterior approach—depends on the condition of the skin and the surgical technique to be used. Its other uses include the following:

1. Drainage of infections in the ankle joint
2. Removal of loose bodies

POSITION OF PATIENT

Place the patient supine on the operating table. Partially exsanguinate the foot either by elevating it for 3 to 5 minutes or by loosely applying a soft rubber bandage to the foot and binding it firmly to the calf. Then inflate a thigh tourniquet. Partial exsanguination allows you to identify the neurovascular bundle, since the venous structures will appear blue. However, you must expect some continuous vascular oozing (Fig. 11-1).

LANDMARKS AND INCISION

Landmarks

The *medial malleolus* is the bulbous subcutaneous distal end of the medial surface of the tibia.

The *lateral malleolus* is the subcutaneous distal end of the fibula.

Incision

Make a 15-cm longitudinal incision over the anterior aspect of the ankle joint. Begin about 10 cm proximal to the joint and extend the incision so that it crosses the joint about midway between the malleoli, ending on the dorsum of the foot. Take great care to cut only the skin; the anterior neurovascular bundle and branches of the superficial peroneal nerve cross the ankle joint very close to the line of the skin incision (Fig. 11-2A).

INTERNERVOUS PLANE

While the approach uses no true internervous plane, the *extensor hallucis longus* and the *extensor digitorum longus* define a clear intermuscular plane. Both muscles are supplied by the deep peroneal nerve, but the plane may be used because both receive their nerve supplies well proximal to the level of the dissection. However, the plane must be used with great caution since it contains the neurovascular bundle distal to the ankle (see Figs. 11-56 and 11-57).

SUPERFICIAL SURGICAL DISSECTION

Incise the deep fascia of the leg in line with the skin incision, cutting through the extensor retinaculum (Fig. 11-2B). Find the plane between the extensor hallucis longus and the extensor digitorum

FIG. 11-1. Position for the anterior approach to the ankle.

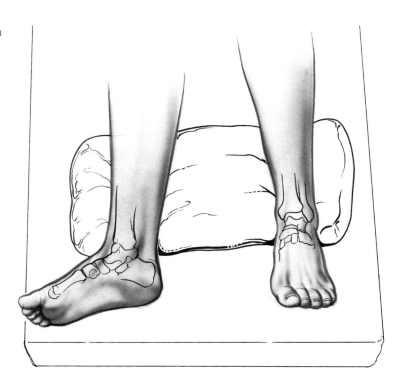

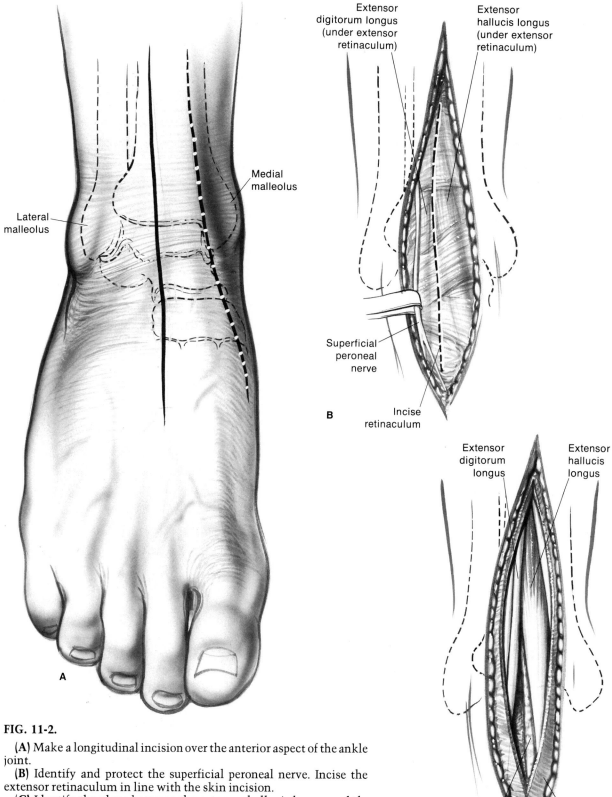

FIG. 11-2.

(**A**) Make a longitudinal incision over the anterior aspect of the ankle joint.

(**B**) Identify and protect the superficial peroneal nerve. Incise the extensor retinaculum in line with the skin incision.

(**C**) Identify the plane between the extensor hallucis longus and the extensor digitorum longus and note the neurovascular bundle between them.

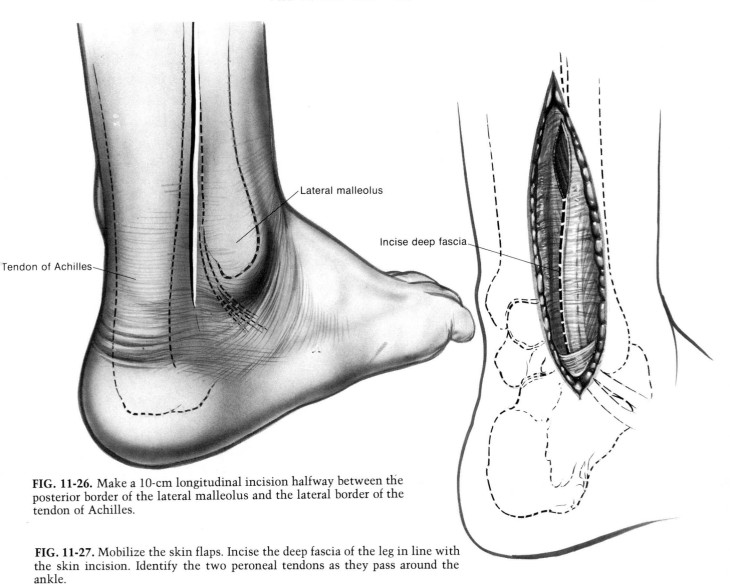

FIG. 11-26. Make a 10-cm longitudinal incision halfway between the posterior border of the lateral malleolus and the lateral border of the tendon of Achilles.

FIG. 11-27. Mobilize the skin flaps. Incise the deep fascia of the leg in line with the skin incision. Identify the two peroneal tendons as they pass around the ankle.

with the skin incision, and identify the two peroneal tendons as they pass down the leg and around the back of the lateral malleolus (Fig. 11-27). The tendon of the peroneus brevis is anterior to that of the peroneus longus at the level of the ankle joint and is, therefore, closer to the lateral malleolus. Note that the peroneus brevis is muscular almost down to the ankle, whereas the peroneus longus is tendinous in the distal third of the leg (see Figs. 11-62 and 11-63).

Incise the peroneal retinaculum to release the tendons, and retract the muscles laterally and anteriorly to expose the flexor hallucis longus (Fig. 11-28). The flexor hallucis longus is the most lateral of the deep flexor muscles of the calf. It is the only one that is still muscular at this level (see Fig. 11-63).

DEEP SURGICAL DISSECTION

To enhance the exposure, make a longitudinal incision through the lateral fibers of the flexor hallucis longus as they arise from the fibula (Fig. 11-29). Retract the flexor hallucis longus medially to reveal the periosteum over the posterior aspect of the tibia (Fig. 11-30). If you have to reach the distal tibia, incise the periosteum longitudinally and strip it medially and laterally to uncover the posterior aspect of the tibia (Fig. 11-31). To enter the ankle joint, follow the posterior aspect of the tibia down to the posterior ankle joint capsule and incise it transversely.

(Text continues on p. 492)

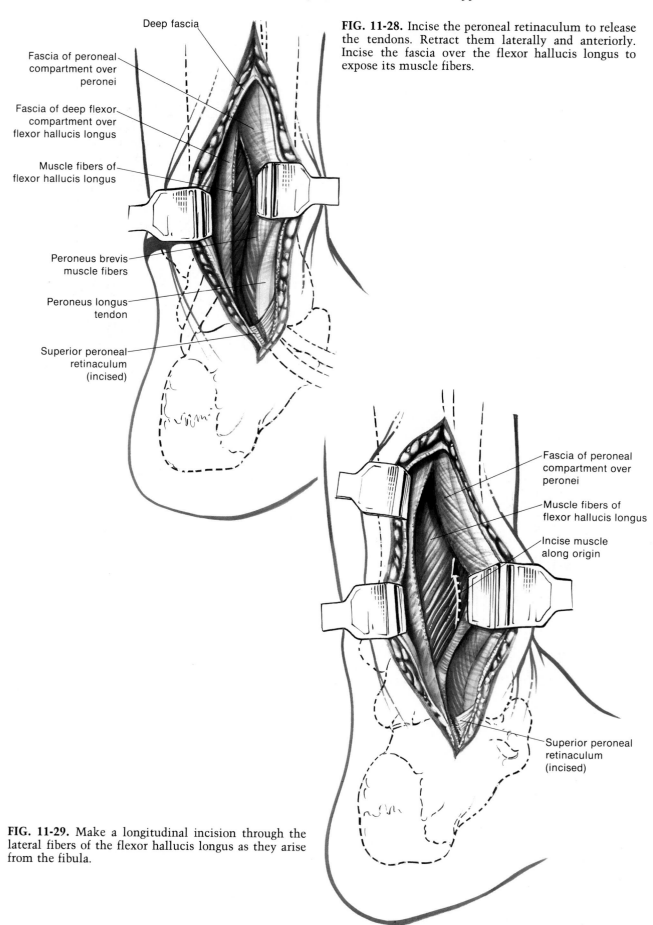

Deep fascia

Fascia of peroneal
compartment over
peronei

Fascia of deep flexor
compartment over
flexor hallucis longus

Muscle fibers of
flexor hallucis longus

Peroneus brevis
muscle fibers

Peroneus longus
tendon

Superior peroneal
retinaculum
(incised)

FIG. 11-28. Incise the peroneal retinaculum to release the tendons. Retract them laterally and anteriorly. Incise the fascia over the flexor hallucis longus to expose its muscle fibers.

Fascia of peroneal
compartment over
peronei

Muscle fibers of
flexor hallucis longus

Incise muscle
along origin

Superior peroneal
retinaculum
(incised)

FIG. 11-29. Make a longitudinal incision through the lateral fibers of the flexor hallucis longus as they arise from the fibula.

LANDMARKS AND INCISION

Landmarks

The *head of the first metatarsal bone* and the *metatarsophalangeal joint* are palpable on the ball of the foot and on its medial border. In cases of bunion, the metatarsal head is medially prominent.

Palpate the *extensor hallucis longus tendon* on the dorsum of the foot. When it is tight, it stands out if you passively plantar flex the great toe.

Incisions

DORSOMEDIAL INCISION: The dorsomedial skin incision gives access to the exostosis on the metatarsal head without much skin retraction; it is by far the most commonly performed incision. It does, however, have its drawbacks: The bursa covering the exostosis may have become inflamed, complicating the surgery, and the skin on the medial aspect of the metatarsophalangeal joint is thinner than on the dorsum of the joint; it may not heal as well.

Begin the dorsomedial incision just proximal to the interphalangeal joint on the dorsomedial aspect of the great toe. Curve it over the dorsal aspect of the metatarsophalangeal joint, keeping medial to the tendon of the extensor hallucis longus. Then curve it back by cutting along the medial aspect of the shaft of the first metatarsal, finishing some 2 cm to 3 cm from the metatarsophalangeal joint (Fig. 11-69).

DORSAL INCISION: Begin the dorsal incision just proximal to the interphalangeal joint and just medial to the tendon of the extensor hallucis longus. Extend the incision proximally, parallel and just medial to the tendon of the extensor hallucis longus. Finish about 2 cm to 3 cm proximal to the metatarsophalangeal joint. Note that the final incision is straight (Fig. 11-72).

INTERNERVOUS PLANE

There is no true internervous plane. The bone is subcutaneous; the two tendons close to the dissection, the extensor hallucis longus and the abductor hallucis, receive their nerve supplies proximal to this approach and cannot be denervated by it.

SUPERFICIAL SURGICAL DISSECTION

Dorsomedial Incision

Incise the deep fascia in line with the incision. Then cut down to the dorsomedial aspect of the metatarsophalangeal joint. The dorsal digital branch of the medial cutaneous nerve, which is often visible, is retracted laterally with the skin flap on the lateral edge of the wound. Make a U-shaped incision into the joint capsule, leaving the capsule attached to the proximal end of the proximal phalanx (Figs. 11-70 and 11-71).

Dorsal Incision

Divide the deep fascia in line with the incision and retract the tendon of the extensor hallucis longus laterally. To enter the joint, incise the dorsal aspect of the joint capsule. Note that the type and position of the capsulotomy depend on the procedure to be performed (Figs. 11-73 and 11-74).

DEEP SURGICAL DISSECTION

For both incisions, incise the periosteum of the proximal phalanx and first metatarsal longitudinally. Using blunt instruments, strip the coverings off the bone, taking care not to damage the tendon of the flexor hallucis longus, which lies in a fibro-osseous tunnel on the plantar surface to the proximal phalanx, between the sesamoids. The extent of the deep dissection depends on the procedure to be carried out. Keep your stripping of periosteum off bone to a minimum. Do not strip all the soft tissue attachments off the metatarsus if you are going to perform a distal osteotomy of that bone, since the metatarsal head is rendered avascular by stripping.

DANGERS

The **tendon of the extensor hallucis longus**, which lies in the lateral edge of the wound, should not be cut during the approach. Indeed, in cases of bunion, the tendon bowstrings laterally across the metatarsophalangeal joint and is even more lateral to the incision than usual. Protect the dorsal digital nerve if you see it along the line of the incision (see Figs. 11-69 and 11-72).

The **tendon of the flexor hallucis longus** is vulnerable as you strip the base of the proximal phalanx. The tendon lies in a groove on the plantar surface of the proximal phalanx so close to the periosteum that, if you are not careful, you may plow into it as you are stripping. The tendon is often displaced laterally in hallux valgus (see Fig. 11-52).

HOW TO ENLARGE THE APPROACH

Careful and systematic stripping of the structures off the bones gives an adequate view of the joint. The approach cannot be usefully extended to other joints in the foot but may be extended proximally for access to the shaft of the metatarsus.

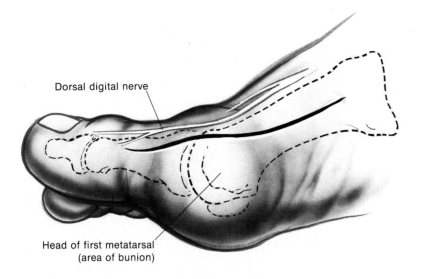

Dorsal digital nerve

Head of first metatarsal
(area of bunion)

FIG. 11-69. Dorsomedial skin incision for the medial approach to the metatarsophalangeal joint of the great toe. Note the proximity of the dorsal digital nerve to the incision.

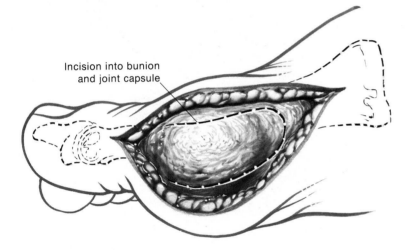

Incision into bunion
and joint capsule

FIG. 11-70. Incise the deep fascia. Develop a joint capsule flap. Protect the dorsal digital branch of the medial cutaneous nerve.

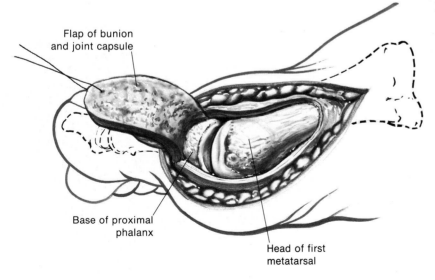

Flap of bunion
and joint capsule

Base of proximal
phalanx

Head of first
metatarsal

FIG. 11-71. Make a U-shaped incision into the joint capsule, leaving the capsule attached to the proximal end of the proximal phalanx.